NOW YOU CAN EAT TO LIVE *AND* LIVE TO EAT!
For diabetics—or anyone who wants to follow a sensible,
healthy diet—this cookbook contains original, delicious
recipes that will appeal to the entire family, including
such tempting favorites as . . .

✳ Cheese Nibblers ✳
✳ Tarragon Soup ✳
✳ Caesar Salad ✳
✳ California Pot Roast ✳
✳ Veal à la King ✳
✳ Charlotte's Curried Chicken ✳
✳ Cranberry Punch ✳
✳ Asparagus with Herbs ✳
✳ Blintzes with Cheese Filling ✳
✳ Date and Nut Bread ✳
✳ Lemon Muffins ✳
✳ Luscious Apricot Soufflé ✳
✳ Chocolate Chiffon Cake with Rum ✳
✳ Strawberry Shortcake ✳

From drinks to desserts and everything in between,
RECIPES FOR DIABETICS offers creative cuisine
everyone will love!

RECIPES
for
DIABETICS

Revised and Updated

by Billie Little

---

preface by
Selvyn B. Bleifer, M.D.

---

revised by
Candace J. Bricker

BANTAM BOOKS

This book is dedicated to the memory of Billie Little from her loving sons, Brian and Bill.
Special thanks to the Bellamys—Freda, Jim, Candace (Bricker), and Jimmy.

The exchange lists are the basis of a meal planning system designed by a committee of the American Diabetes Association and The American Dietetic Association. While designed primarily for people with diabetes and others who must follow special diets, the exchange lists are based on principles of good nutrition that apply to everyone. Copyright © 1986 by the American Diabetes Association, The American Dietetic Association.

This book is not intended to replace your own physician, with whom you should consult before embarking on any new diet program.

RECIPES FOR DIABETICS
A Bantam Book published by arrangement with The Putnam Publishing Group

PUBLISHING HISTORY
Grosset & Dunlap edition published March 1972
Bantam edition / July 1975
Grosset revised edition / June 1981
Bantam revised and updated edition / September 1985
GD/Perigee Books revised and updated edition published 1990
Bantam second revised and updated edition / October 1991
Perigee revised and updated edition / May 1999
Bantam revised and updated edition / November 2001
Bantam reissue / September 2007

Published by Bantam Dell
A Division of Random House, Inc.
New York, New York

Library of Congress Catalog Card Number: 98-53075

ISBN 978-0-553-58472-1

Printed in the United States of America
Published simultaneously in Canada

www.bantamdell.com

OPM   16

CONTENTS

FOREWORD

These recipes are intended to help and guide you in preparing and serving attractive, colorful, unusual, and satisfying meals while conforming to your diabetic diet.

It is important that you follow your doctor's diet orders explicitly and use only those recipes suited to your particular suggested calorie intake.

The variety of recipes offered is intended to stimulate your interest in following your diet strictly, proving that your diet need not be monotonous and unappetizing. Many of these recipes can also be enjoyed by the entire family.

PREFACE

There are, by conservative estimates, approximately 20 million diabetics in the United States today. Sophisticated studies could detect millions more who are frankly diabetic or destined to develop diabetes.

Treatment varies depending upon the age of the patient and severity of the diabetes. In every case, diet is the key to the treatment, and a majority of diabetics may be treated by diet alone.

Even in patients whose treatment requires insulin and/or oral agents, diet is as important as the drugs. Most diabetics are overweight and should, as part of the treatment, exercise and restrict calories.

The American public is confused by a plethora of books on diet. Diets to lose weight; diets to lower the serum cholesterol; special diets for people with kidney failure, kidney stones, or gout; or special diets that are high in fiber or high in protein.

Your doctor will prescribe the proper diet (total calories, protein, and fat content), as well as the proper amount of exercise. In addition, insulin or oral diabetic drugs may be prescribed.

Diabetics who develop the disease after 50 years of age are classified as adult onset or maturity onset diabetics or Type II diabetics. The vast majority of Type II patients may be treated by diet alone—with exercise but without drugs.

Recipes for Diabetics by Billie Little addresses the needs of diabetics by providing a book that is easy to understand and including wonderful recipes that are simple and easy to prepare.

There is nothing different or special about recipes for diabetics. Anyone who desires to lose weight or go on a balanced nutrition diet should find this book ideal.

This new edition is more complete and informative and

should be in the kitchen of every woman (or man) concerned
with proper nutrition, especially in diabetic families.

SELVYN B. BLEIFER, M.D., F.A.C.P., F.A.C.C.
Associate Clinical Professor of Medicine,
UCLA Medical School
Torrance, California

ACKNOWLEDGMENTS

So very many friends, relatives, and diabetic patients have contributed their ideas and treasured recipes that we wish to give a special note of thanks to them and to the food companies, firms, newspapers, and magazines whose information appears in this book. We gratefully acknowledge permission from the following:

Adolphs, 5355 Cartwright, North Hollywood, CA 91601

Alba Foods (skim milk products), 800 Third Ave., New York, NY 10020

Batter Lite Foods (fructose, Batter Lite cake batters, etc.), P.O. Box 321, Beloit, WI 53511

Beatrice Foods, 1526 South State St., Chicago, IL 69605

Borden Inc. (Lite Line cheeses), 180 E. Broad St., 25th Floor, P.O. Box 40789, Columbus, OH 43201

Campbell Soup Company, Campbell Place, Camden, NJ 08103-1701

Carnation Foods, c/o Nestle Food Co., Glendale, CA 91203

Cumberland Packing Co. (Sweet'n Low Division), 2 Cumberland St., Brooklyn, NY 11205. (Butter Buds), 1636 Taylor, Racine, WI 53403

Diet & Health Products (Fisher Cheese Co.), P.O. Box 1886, Lima, OH 45802

Eli Lilly & Company, Indianapolis, IN 46206

Food and Nutrition Board, 2101 Constitution Ave., Washington, DC 20418

Frito-Lay, Inc., 7701 Legacy Drive, Plano, TX 75024

General Mills Chemicals, Inc., 4620 W. 77th St., Minneapolis, MN 55435. (Yoplait), P.O. Box 1113, Minneapolis, MN 55440

Good Food Unit #306, National Health Systems—The Times, P.O. Box 1501, Ann Arbor, MI 48106

Haddon House, Marlton Pike, Medford, NJ 08055

Henkel Corp. (dietary specialties), 4620 W. 7th St., Minneapolis, MN 55435

Knox Gelatin, Inc., 800 Sylvan Ave., Englewood Cliffs, NJ 07632

Kraft Foods, Inc., Glenview, IL 60025

Lever Brothers, New York, NY 10022

M C P Foods (Slim Set, mix for jams and jellies), P.O. Box 3633, Anaheim, CA 92803

National Dairy Council, 6300 North River Rd., Rosemont, IL 60018

National Health Systems, P.O. Box 1501, Ann Arbor, MI 48106

Pillsbury Company (Sprinkle Sweet), 311 2nd St., S.E.; Minneapolis, MN 55414

Plough, Inc. (Ril Sweet), Memphis, TN 38101

Rosarita Products (low-calorie Mexican foods), c/o Hunt Wesson, Inc., P.O. Box 4800, Fullerton, CA 92834

Specialty Brands, Inc. (Spice Islands, Marie's Refrigerated Dressings), a Division of Burns Philip Foods, Inc., San Francisco, CA 94108

Spreckels Sugar Co. (sugar products), 121 Spreckels Blvd., Salinas, CA 93901

Sterling Food Co. (soya, carob flour mix), 5118 Fourteenth Ave. N.W., Seattle, WA 98107

Sugar Lo (Parv-A-Zert, frozen dietetic desserts), 2001 Bacharach Blvd., Atlantic City, NJ 08401, Attn: Alan E. Kligerman

Superose Sweetener, G. H. Whitlock Process Co., P.O. Box 259, Springfield, IL 62705

Sweet'n Natural (Sweet'n Natural fruit sugar), P.O. Box 55086, Sherman Oaks, CA 91403; or P.O. Box 410, Brooklyn, NY 11202

Tillie Lewis Foods, Inc. (low-calorie foods), P.O. Drawer J, Stockton, CA 95201

Thomas J. Lipton, Inc. (Wish-Bone Lite and other low-calorie salad dressings), 800 Sylvan Ave., Englewood Cliffs, NJ 07632

Tropicana Products, Inc. (pure orange juice), P.O. Box 338, Bradenton, FL 33506

U.S. Government

Department of Agriculture, Agricultural Research Service, Independence Ave., 12th & 14th Sts. S.W., Washington, DC 20251

Department of Agriculture, Science & Education Administration, Consumer & Food Economic Institute, Hyattsville, MD 20782

Department of Health and Human Services, Public Health Service, Food & Drug Administration, Consumer Communications Staff, 5600 Fishers Lane HFJ, Rockville, MD 20857

SPECIAL THANKS TO: Miss Carol Edgar, Public Relations Division, Eli Lilly and Company, Indianapolis, IN, for her assistance and permission to use information contained in the many excellent booklets distributed by this fine company; to Mr. James R. Schmidt of Tillie Lewis; to the Public Health Service and other government sources; to Mary Helen Gunkler, R.D., Nutrition Department, General Mills, Inc.; and last but not least to Marie Slavens, our typist, for patiently wading through our notes.

Additional information on medication, reactions, travel and vacation, food care, and so on will be found in "Diabetes and You," available from the Superintendent of Documents, U.S. Government Printing Office, Washington, DC 20402. Also refer to the section on Printed Material Available at the back of this book for booklets, books, and other pertinent information that can be obtained for little or no charge.

REMEMBER

While many people (in addition to your doctor)—a dietitian or nurse, for example—can assist you in learning to control diabetes, it is up to *you* to:

1. Continue under medical supervision.
2. Use the exact amount and type of medication prescribed for you! Follow this plan, paying special attention to precise amounts and kinds of food and the time schedule prescribed for you by your doctor.
3. Use the exact diet plan worked out for you.
4. Do some exercise in the same amounts, each day. (The latest information we have is that the right exercise helps produce the amount of insulin a diabetic needs. Consult your physician for *your* proper exercise program.)
5. In addition to your regular physical checkup, have a regular eye examination, *especially* if you are being treated with insulin; the American Association of Ophthalmologists reports that "about 12 percent of all new blindness in the United States is due to complications of diabetes."
6. Practice good habits of personal hygiene to minimize the possibility of infection.

WEIGHTS, MEASURES, AND THE METRIC SYSTEM

The care provider who is planning meals for a diabetic needs to know something about food values. The following tables will help determine measurements for carbohydrates, fats, and proteins. Also included are equivalents for most of the measures used in these tables. Be sure to use standard measuring utensils, such as an 8-ounce measuring cup, tablespoon, teaspoon, and the like. (Drug and discount stores also carry a set of measuring spoons covering sizes from ⅛ teaspoon to 1 tablespoon.) It is also a good idea to remeasure after cooking. There are a few foods that need not be measured; these are noted in the Exchange Lists.

EVERYDAY WEIGHTS AND MEASURES

3 teaspoons	1 tablespoon
2 tablespoons	⅛ cup
4 tablespoons	¼ cup
5 tablespoons + 1 teaspoon	⅓ cup
8 tablespoons	½ cup
12 tablespoons	¾ cup
16 tablespoons	1 cup
2 cups	1 pint
2 pints	1 quart
4 quarts	1 gallon
1 fluid ounce	12 tablespoons
16 ounces	1 pound
1 pound butter or margarine	4 sticks, 2 cups, or 64 pats or squares
1 stick butter	½ cup (approximate) or 16 pats or squares
Dash or "few grains"	up to ⅛ teaspoon

METRIC SYSTEM

Liquid Measure

The metric system is based on units of 10. For liquid measure, the simple metric unit is the liter, which is just a little larger than our quart. One teaspoon is equivalent to 5 milliliters (or 5 cubic centimeters—a unit that drug dispensers prefer).

Units of Measure

1 milliliter = 1 cubic centimeter
1000 milliliters = 1 liter

Equivalents

1 teaspoon = 5 milliliters
1 tablespoon = 15 milliliters
1 cup = 0.24 liter
1 pint = 0.47 liter
1 quart = 0.946 liter
1 gallon = 3.8 liters
1 fluid ounce = 29.57 milliliters

Unit Conversion

To convert	into	multiply by
gallons	liters	3.785
liters	gallons	0.264
liters	pints	2.113
quarts	liters	0.946

The boiling point of water is: 212.0° Fahrenheit, or 100° Celsius or Centigrade.

Dry Measure

The basic unit of metric weight is the gram; this unit is approximately one-thirtieth of an avoirdupois ounce and is mostly used in pharmaceutical and scientific work. The more convenient unit is the kilogram, weighing approximately 2.2 pounds.

Units of Measure
1000 milligrams = 1 gram
100 centigrams = 1 gram
1000 grams = 1 kilogram

Equivalents
1 ounce = 28.35 grams
1 pound = 0.45 kilograms
2.2 pounds = 1 kilogram

Unit Conversion

To convert	into	multiply by
grams	ounces	0.035
grams	pounds	0.002
ounces	grams	28.35
pounds	kilograms	0.454

Calories

1 gram carbohydrate	4 calories
1 gram fat	9 calories
1 gram protein	4 calories
1 cup nondairy whip	160 calories (approximately)

Examples: 1 teaspoon sugar is 5 grams carbohydrate
(20 calories)
1 teaspoon margarine or butter is 5 grams fat
(45 calories)

GENERAL RULES

MEASURING FOOD

Most foods should be measured. You will need a standard 8-ounce measuring cup, measuring teaspoon, and tablespoon, and an ounce or gram scale. All measurements are level. Most foods are measured after cooking.

Careful measurement is more important for meat and fat quantities than for fruit, juices, and starches. Careful measuring of vegetables is less important as they generally are low in calories and fat.

It is important to measure foods at the beginning so you become acquainted with real serving sizes. (However, it really isn't necessary for you to weigh every bean!)

FOOD PREPARATION

Meats may be baked, boiled, roasted or broiled (indoors or on an outdoor grill). Do not fry foods except in fat exchanges allowed for that meal. Vegetables may be prepared with the family meals, but the portion for the diabetic should be removed before extra fat exchanges or bread exchanges are added. Fat allowed in your diet may be used to season vegetables. Vegetables may be cooked in bouillon or fat-free meat broth if desired.

SPECIAL FOODS

It is not necessary to buy special foods. Select the diet from the same foods purchased for the rest of the family—milk, vegetables, bread, meats, fats, and fruit (fresh, dried, or canned without sugar). "Special dietetic foods" should be used with discretion; always check the labels of these foods for protein, carbohydrate, fat, and calorie content. Be sure additional calories in special diet foods are figured in the diet.

NOTE: Scientific tests indicate that saccharin may be dangerous to your health and, taken in large quantities, may be cancer causing. Its use is cautioned because of its ability to cause cancer in experimental animals.

FREE FOODS

Seasonings: Cinnamon, celery salt, garlic, garlic salt, lemon, mustard, mint, nutmeg, parsley, pepper, sugarless sweeteners, spices, vanilla, and vinegar. *Other foods:* Coffee or tea (without sugar or cream), fat-free broth, bouillon, unflavored gelatin, sour or dill pickles, cranberries (with nonnutritive sweetener or sugar substitute).

FOODS TO AVOID

Beer, wine, and other alcoholic beverages.

Sugar. New research shows that all carbohydrates are digested at about the same speed. Whether the carbohydrate is simple (like sugar) or complex (like bread) doesn't matter. Both kinds raise your glucose levels at about the same rate.

For this reason, sugar is no longer a no-no. But you must work it into your food plan in place of other carbohydrates. Ask your dietitian to show you how.

Also, keep in mind that sugar has calories but no vitamins. Foods with sugar often have fat as well. The American Diabetes Association considers some artificial sweeteners safe in moderate amounts. These include saccharin, aspartame (Nutra-Sweet), and acesulfame potassium (Sweet One).

EXCHANGE LISTS

SPECIAL NOTE:
Negligible (trace) and less than ⅙ exchanges are
not figured in the recipes in this book.
Calories are rounded off.

The following pages and the recipes in this book are based on the 1995 version of the *Exchange Lists for Meal Planning*.

Your registered dietitian or doctor will select items from the following food groups according to their carbohydrate, fat, and protein content, calorie count, and so on. To ensure good nutrition, your diet should include the same essential foods, sometimes referred to as the "basic six," recommended for everyone:

1. Milk
2. Vegetables
3. Fruits
4. Starches (cereals, bread, starchy vegetables)
5. Meat
6. Fat

Foods on the same list have about the same nutritional value. The groupings are called "exchange lists" because one food may be exchanged for another on the same list, *but* foods on one list may *not* be exchanged for foods on another list. Each diet plan includes foods from all exchange lists to give variety.

The diabetic person on a rigid restricted-calorie diet should avoid too many bread, fat, and meat exchanges. The calorie counts and exchanges have been calculated from the diabetic exchange lists found on the next few pages. Different exchange groupings vary slightly. It is imperative that a diabetic follow the calorie prescription given him or her by the doctor and the exchange lists that are included with his or her own diet order.

(A strict diabetic should recalculate these recipes if using a different exchange system.) Different methods of recipe preparation, interpretation of ingredients, types of nonnutritive sweeteners (both liquid and granulated), and so on, will vary the volume of the recipe and approximate yield. If the yield is different, the calories of the recipe need to be recalculated, and the exchanges refigured.

EXCHANGE LISTS
FOR MEAL PLANNING

The exchange lists are the basis of a meal planning system designed by a committee of the American Diabetes Association and The American Dietetic Association. While designed primarily for people with diabetes and others who must follow special diets, the exchange lists are based on principles of good nutrition that apply to everyone. Copyright © 1986 American Diabetes Association, The American Dietetic Association.

An "exchange" is a measured *portion* of food. The size or quantity of each exchange on the list is already developed for you in easy household measurements.

One of the most important aspects of diabetes management is dietary care. The food exchanges are lists of foods grouped by similar values of carbohydrates, proteins, and fats so that one food can be substituted for another in your daily meal plans. Foods have been divided into six categories—milks, vegetables, fruits, breads, meats, and fats. Foods in any one group can be substituted or exchanged with other foods *within the same group*.

We suggest that you consult your physician or nutritionist about your meal plan. You will be told how many exchanges you can have from each of the six lists, taking into account how many calories will be best for you. The number of calories will be based on your health, energy needs, and physical activities.

Eat only those foods on the diet list. Eat only the amounts of food shown. Do not skip meals. Do not eat between meals.

List #1: Milk Exchanges:

Based on the amount of fat they contain, milks are divided into skim/very low-fat milk, low-fat milk, and whole milk. One choice of these includes:

	Carbohydrate (grams)	Protein (grams)	Fat (grams)	Calories
Skim/very low-fat	12	8	0–3	90
Low-fat	12	8	5	120
Whole	12	8	8	150

Skim and Very Low-Fat Milk   QUANTITY

Skim or nonfat milk	1 cup
½% milk	1 cup
1% milk	1 cup
Dry nonfat milk	⅓ cup dry
Canned, evaporated skim milk	½ cup
Lowfat buttermilk	1 cup
Plain nonfat yogurt	¾ cup
Nonfat or low-fat fruit-flavored yogurt sweetened with aspartame or with a nonnutritive sweetener	1 cup

Low-Fat Milk   QUANTITY

2% milk	1 cup
Plain low-fat yogurt	¾ cup
Sweet acidophilus milk	1 cup

Whole Milk   QUANTITY

Whole milk	1 cup
Evaporated whole milk	½ cup
Goat's milk	1 cup
Kefir	1 cup

List #2: Vegetable Exchanges:

One Exchange of Vegetables contains about 5 grams of carbohydrate, 2 grams of protein, and 25 calories. One Exchange also provides 1–4 grams of dietary fiber. One Exchange is one cup of raw vegetables or ½ cup cooked or juiced vegetables.

Artichoke (½ medium)
Asparagus
Beans (green, wax, Italian)
Bean sprouts
Beets
Broccoli
Brussels sprouts
Cabbage
Carrots
Cauliflower
Celery
Cucumber
Eggplant
Green onion
Green (collards, mustard, turnips)
Kohlrabi
Leeks
Mixed vegetables (without corn, peas, or pasta)
Mushrooms
Okra
Onions
Pea pods
Peppers (all varieties)
Radishes
Salad greens (endive, escarole, lettuce, romaine, spinach)
Sauerkraut
Spinach
Summer squash (crookneck)
Tomato
Tomatoes, canned
Tomato sauce
Tomato/vegetable juice
Turnips
Water chestnuts
Watercress
Zucchini

Starchy vegetables such as corn, peas, and potatoes are found on the Starch/Bread Exchange List.

List #3: Fruit Exchanges:
One Exchange of Fruit contains 15 grams of carbohydrate and 60 calories.

NOTE: One serving of fresh fruit contains 2 grams of fiber.

Apple	1 (4 oz.)	Blackberries (raw)	¾ cup
Applesauce, unsweetened	½ cup	Blueberries (raw)	¾ cup
		Cantaloupe	⅓ small
Apricots, fresh	4 medium (5½ oz.)		(11 oz. or 1 cup cubes)
Apricots (canned)	½ cup	Cherries, fresh	12 large
Banana	1 (4 oz.)	Cherries (canned)	½ cup

Figs (raw)	2 medium (3½ oz.)	Pear (raw)	½ large or 1 small
Fruit cocktail (canned)	½ cup	Pears (canned)	½ cup or 2 halves
Grapefruit	½ large (11 oz.)	Persimmon	2 medium
Grapefruit (sections)	¾ cup	Pineapple (raw)	¾ cup
Grapes	17 small (3 oz.)	Pineapple (canned)	½ cup
Honeydew melon	1 slice (10 oz.) or 1 cup cubes	Plum (raw)	2 small (5 oz.)
		Plum (canned)	½ cup
Kiwi	1 large	Pomegranate	½ fruit
Mandarin oranges	¾ cup	Raspberries (raw)	1 cup
Mango	½ small or ½ cup	Strawberries (raw, whole)	1¼ cups
Nectarine	1 small (5 oz.)		
Orange	1 small (6½ oz.)	Tangerine	2 small (8 oz.)
Papaya	½ fruit or 1 cup cubes	Watermelon	1 slice (13½ oz.) or 1¼ cups cubes
Peach (raw)	1 medium (6 oz.)		

Dried Fruit:			
Apples	4 rings	Figs	1½
Apricots	8 halves	Prunes	3 medium
Dates	3 medium	Raisins	2 Tbsp.

Fruit Juice:		Fruit juice blends,	
Apple juice/cider	½ cup	100% juice	⅓ cup
Cranberry juice cocktail	⅓ cup	Grapefruit juice	½ cup
		Grape juice	⅓ cup
Cranberry juice cocktail, reduced-calorie	1 cup	Orange juice	½ cup
		Pineapple juice	½ cup
		Prune Juice	⅓ cup

List #4: Starch Exchanges:

One Exchange of Starch contains 15 grams of carbohydrate, 3 grams of protein, 0–1 gram of fat, and 80 calories.

NOTE: In general, one Starch is ½ cup of cereal, grain, pasta, or starchy vegetable; 1 ounce of bread product, such as 1 slice of bread; and ¾ to 1 ounce of most snack foods. (Some snack foods may also have added fat.) Wherever possible, choose foods made from whole grains, which are good sources of fiber. Beans, peas, and lentils are a good source of protein and fiber.

Bread:

Bagel	½ (1 oz.)
Bread, reduced-calorie	2 slices (1½ oz.)
Bread, white, whole wheat, pumpernickel, rye	1 slice (1 oz.)
Bread sticks, crisp, 4″ × ½″	2 (⅔ oz.)
English muffin	½
Hot dog or hamburger bun	½ (1 oz.)
Pita, 6″ across	½
Raisin bread, unfrosted	1 slice (1 oz.)
Roll, plain, small	1 (1 oz.)
Tortilla, corn, 6″ across	1
Tortilla, flour, 7–8″ across	1
Waffle, 4½″ square reduced-fat	1

Cereals/Grains/Pasta:

Bran cereals, concentrated	⅓ cup
Bran cereals, flaked	½ cup
Bulgur (cooked)	½ cup
Cereals (cooked)	½ cup
Cereals, unsweetened, ready-to-eat	¾ cup
Cornmeal (dry)	3 Tbsp.
Couscous	⅓ cup
Flour (dry)	3 Tbsp.
Granola, low-fat	¼ cup
Grape-Nuts	¼ cup
Grits	½ cup
Kasha	½ cup
Millet	¼ cup
Meusli	¼ cup
Oats	½ cup
Pasta (cooked)	½ cup
Puffed cereal	1½ cups
Rice milk	½ cup
Rice, white or brown	⅓ cup
Shredded wheat	½ cup
Sugar-frosted cereal	½ cup
Wheat germ	3 Tbsp.

Crackers/Snacks:

Animal crackers	8
Graham crackers, 2½″ square	3
Matzoh	¾ oz.
Melba toast	4 slices
Oyster crackers	24
Popcorn (popped, no fat added or low-fat microwave)	3 cups
Pretzels	¾ oz.
Rice cakes, 4″ across	2
Saltine-type crackers	6
Snack chips, fat-free	15–20
Whole wheat crackers, no fat added	2–5 (3–5 oz.)

Starchy Vegetables:

Baked beans	⅓ cup
Corn	½ cup
Corn on cob, medium	1 (5 oz.)
Lentils	½ cup
Lima beans	⅔ cup
Miso	3 Tbsp.
Mixed vegetables with corn, peas, or pasta	1 cup
Peas, green	½ cup
Plantain	½ cup
Potato, baked or broiled	1 small (3 oz.)
Potato, mashed	½ cup
Squash, winter (acorn, butternut)	1 cup
Yam, sweet potato, plain	½ cup

STARCH FOODS PREPARED WITH FAT:

(Count as 1 Starch Exchange, plus 1 Fat Exchange)

Biscuit, 2½″ across	1
Chow mein noodles	½ cup
Corn bread, 2″ cube	1 (2 oz.)
Crackers, round butter type	6
Croutons	1 cup
French fried potatoes	16–25 (3 oz.)
Granola	¼ cup
Muffin, small	1 (1½ oz.)
Pancake, 4″ across	2
Popcorn, microwave	3 cups
Sandwich crackers, cheese or peanut butter filling	3
Stuffing, bread (prepared)	⅓ cup
Taco shell, 6″ across	2
Waffle, 4½″ square	1
Whole wheat crackers, fat added	4–6

List #5: Meat and Meat Substitutes:

In general, one Meat Exchange is 1 oz. meat, fish, poultry, or cheese; ½ cup beans, peas, or lentils. Based upon the amount of fat they contain, meats are divided into Very Lean, Lean, Medium-Fat, and High-Fat lists. This is done so you can see which ones contain the least amount of fat. One ounce (one exchange) of each of these includes:

	Carbohydrate (grams)	Protein (grams)	Fat (grams)	Calories
Very Lean	0	7	0–1	35
Lean	0	7	3	55
Medium-Fat	0	7	5	75
High-Fat	0	7	8	100

VERY LEAN MEAT:

Poultry:	Chicken or turkey (white meat, no skin), Cornish hen (no skin)	1 oz.
Fish:	Fresh or frozen cod, flounder, haddock, halibut, trout; tuna (fresh or canned in water)	1 oz.
Shellfish:	Clams, crab, lobster, scallops, shrimp, imitation shellfish	1 oz.
Game:	Duck or pheasant (no skin), venison, buffalo, ostrich	1 oz.

Cheese with 1 gram or less fat per ounce:

	Nonfat or low-fat cottage cheese	¼ cup
	Fat-free cheese	1 oz.
Other:	Processed sandwich meats with 1 gram or less fat per ounce, such as deli thin, shaved meats, chipped beef, turkey ham	1 oz.
	Egg whites	2
	Egg substitutes, plain	¼ cup
	Hot dogs with 1 gram or less fat per ounce	1 oz.
	Kidney (high in cholesterol)	1 oz.

Sausage with 1 gram or less fat per ounce	1 oz.
Beans, peas, lentils (cooked)—count as one	
Very Lean Meat and one Starch Exchange	½ cup

LEAN MEAT:

Beef: USDA Select or Choice grades of lean beef trimmed of fat, such as round, sirloin, flank, (T-bone, porterhouse, and cubed) steak; tenderloin; roast (rib, chuck, rump); ground round   1 oz.

Pork: Lean pork, such as fresh ham; canned, cured, or boiled ham; Canadian bacon; tenderloin, center loin chop   1 oz.

Lamb: Roast, chop, leg   1 oz.

Veal: Lean chop, roast   1 oz.

Poultry: Chicken, turkey (dark meat, no skin), chicken (white meat, with skin), domestic duck or goose (well-drained of fat, no skin)   1 oz.

Fish: Herring (uncreamed or smoked)   1 oz.
Oysters   6 medium
Salmon (fresh or canned), catfish   1 oz.
Sardines (canned)   2 medium
Tuna (canned in oil, drained)   1 oz.

Game: Goose (no skin), rabbit   1 oz.

Cheese: 4.5% fat cottage cheese   ¼ cup
Grated Parmesan   2 Tbsp.
Cheeses with 3 grams or less fat per ounce   1 oz.

Other: Hot dogs with 3 grams or less fat per ounce   1½ oz.
Processed sandwich meat with 3 grams or less fat per ounce, such as turkey pastrami or kielbasa   1 oz.
Liver, heart (high in cholesterol)   1 oz.

MEDIUM-FAT MEAT:

Beef: Most beef products fall into this category (ground beef, meatloaf, corned beef,

	short ribs, prime grades of meat trimmed of fat, such as prime rib)	1 oz.
Pork:	Top loin, chop, Boston butt, cutlet	1 oz.
Lamb:	Rib roast, ground	1 oz.
Veal:	Cutlet (ground or cubed, unbreaded)	1 oz.
Poultry:	Chicken (dark meat, with skin), ground turkey or ground chicken, fried chicken (with skin)	1 oz.
Fish:	Any fried fish product	1 oz.
Cheese:	With 5 grams or less fat per ounce	
	Feta	1 oz.
	Mozzarella	1 oz.
	Ricotta	¼ cup (2 oz.)
Other:	Egg (high in cholesterol, limit to 3 per week)	1
	Sausage with 5 grams or less fat per ounce	1 oz.
	Soy milk	1 cup
	Tempeh	¼ cup
	Tofu	4 oz. or ½ cup

HIGH-FAT MEAT: Remember, these items are high in saturated fat, cholesterol, and calories and may raise blood cholesterol levels if eaten on a regular basis.

Pork:	Spareribs, ground pork, pork sausage	1 oz.
Cheese:	All regular cheeses, such as American, cheddar, Monterey Jack, Swiss	1 oz.
Other:	Processed sandwich meats with 8 grams or less fat per ounce, such as bologna, pimento loaf, salami	1 oz.
	Sausage, such as bratwurst, Italian, knockwurst, Polish, smoked	1 oz.
	Hot dog (turkey or chicken)	1 (10/lb.)
	Bacon	3 slices (20 slices/lb.)
	Hot dog (beef, pork, or combination)— count as one High-Fat Meat plus one Fat Exchange	1(10/lb.)

Peanut butter (contains unsaturated fat)—
count as one High-Fat Meat plus two
Fat Exchanges 2 Tbsp.

List #6: Fat Exchanges:

Fats are divided into three groups, based on the main type of fat they contain: monounsaturated, polyunsaturated, and saturated. Small amounts of monounsaturated and polyunsaturated fats in the foods we eat are linked with good health benefits. Saturated fats are linked with heart disease and cancer. One Fat Exchange contains 5 grams of fat and 45 calories.

Monounsaturated

Avocado, medium ⅛ (1 oz.)		Olives: ripe (black)	8 large
Nuts:		green, stuffed	10 large
Almonds, cashews	6 nuts	Peanut butter: smooth	
Mixed (50% peanuts)		or crunchy	2 tsp.
	6 nuts	Sesame seeds	1 Tbsp.
Peanuts	10 nuts	Tahini paste	2 tsp.
Pecans	4 halves		
Oil (canola, olive, peanut)	1 tsp.		

Polyunsaturated

Margarine: stick, tub, or squeeze	1 tsp.	Salad dressing: regular	1 Tbsp.
Lower-fat (30%–50% vegetable oil)	1 Tbsp.	reduced-fat	2 Tbsp.
Mayonnaise: regular		Miracle Whip Salad Dressing: regular	2 tsp.
reduced-fat	1 tsp.	reduced-fat	1 Tbsp.
Nuts: walnuts, English	4 halves	Seeds: pumpkin, sunflower	1 Tbsp.
Oil (corn, safflower, soybean)	1 tsp.		

Saturated

Bacon, cooked	1 slice (20 slices/lb.)	Coffee whitener, powder	4 tsp.
Bacon, grease	1 tsp.	Cream, half-and-half	2 Tbsp.
Butter: stick	1 tsp.	Cream cheese:	
whipped	2 tsp.	regular	1 Tbsp.
reduced-fat	1 Tbsp.	reduced-fat	2 Tbsp.
Chitterlings, boiled	2 Tbsp. (½ oz.)	Salt pork	¼ oz.
		Shortening or lard	1 tsp.
Coconut, sweetened, shredded	2 Tbsp.	Sour cream:	
Coffee whitener, liquid	2 Tbsp.	regular	2 Tbsp.
		reduced-fat	3 Tbsp.

NOTES ON SPECIAL INGREDIENTS USED IN RECIPES

1. In order to reduce the caloric content of numerous recipes without affecting quality, we have included various diet ingredients available in local supermarkets. We have calculated the calories and exchange groupings in our recipes using the following diet products:

   diet margarine
   diet mayonnaise
   diet salad dressings
   imitation dairy and nondairy products
   diet puddings
   diet sauces and toppings

   If you prefer to use an ingredient other than the diet supplement, you will have to adjust the calories and exchanges.

2. Sweeteners: No-calorie sweeteners may be substituted for sugar in many recipes, and also used on foods that need a certain amount of sweetening. They are sold in granulated, liquid, and tablet form. Granulated sweetener may be sprinkled on cereals and fresh fruits; it dissolves immediately. For cold beverages the liquid is most convenient, and either the tablet or the granulated form may be used in cooking or in hot beverages. For best results, add the sweetening agent toward the end of the cooking process, since the sweetening power is lessened when exposed to high or low temperatures for a long period of time.

   Sweeteners are available with either a calcium or a sodium base. Calcium-based sweeteners are slightly less sweet than the sodium forms. They are suggested for the diabetic who is on a low-sodium diet.

If you find too much substitute has been used, and that it leaves a bitter taste in your mouth, counteract it with a little salt (if it is permitted in your diet).

The many sugar substitutes on the market include Equal, Fructose, Nectasweet, NutraSweet, Sugartwin, Sweet Lite (Fructose), Sweet'n Low, and Sweet One. There are also others, which you may prefer.

For *Substitute Sugar Syrup*, combine equal quantities of water and sugar substitute. Bring to a boil; boil 5 minutes or so. Store in a covered jar in your refrigerator and use for sweetening cold drinks. (This may be used in place of the commercial liquid sweetener.)

SYRUPS: (May be used to sweeten fruits for canning.)

Light: 7 teaspoons of sugar substitute and 4 cups of water. Boil together 5 minutes. Skim. Makes 4½ cups.

Medium: 3 teaspoons substitute, 3 cups water. Boil 5 minutes. Skim. Makes approximately 3 cups.

Heavy: 20 teaspoons substitute, 2 cups water. Boil 5 minutes. Skim. Makes 2⅔ cups.

GLAZES: Nonnutritive sweetener equivalent to 1 cup brown sugar, juice and grated rind of 1 orange.

Nonnutritive sweetener equivalent to 1 cup sugar, ½ cup cider, dietetic maraschino cherry juice, or sweet pickle juice.

½ cup (4 ounces) dietetic currant jelly, melted.

½ cup dietetic orange marmalade, softened.

There are several brown sugar substitutes available, but if you cannot locate any and brown sugar is called for in a recipe, put granulated white sugar substitute in a frying pan over *very low heat;* stir constantly until caramelized.

Use bulk nonnutritives for baked goods, such as cakes, cookies, and bread. For drinks, use liquid nonnutritive sweeteners.

Liquid sweeteners are used by the drop. For example: ½ cup of granulated regular sugar, or granulated sugar substitute, is the equivalent of 1 tablespoon of liquid sweetener.

3. All diet margarines contain fewer than half the calories of regular margarine—17 calories per teaspoon, 50 calories per tablespoon. Although diet margarine is not recommended for frying, it can, with proper care, be used (first melt *slowly* in a frying pan; add food, cover, and cook over *low* heat). When baking, remember that it has only half the fat content of regular margarine; so, since tampering with the fat content of baked goods can ruin the finished products, we suggest using the regular soft-form or stick-form margarines in recipes calling for more than 2 tablespoons of margarine.

4. WINE AND LIQUOR NOTES. The recipes containing alcohol are not for diabetics without explicit consent of their own doctor. Each recipe containing beer, liqueurs, liquor, or wine is specially marked.

5. PURE ORANGE JUICE NOTE. Remember that pure orange juice contains approximately 11–12 percent natural fruit sugars; consult your physician about using it.

AIDS TO VARYING MEALS

Bake, broil, or roast meats. Bake, broil, or poach fish.

Add herbs to meat and vegetables. Use ¼ teaspoon dry herbs for each 6 servings of fish, meat, or vegetables. Try basil, rosemary, garlic salt, dry mustard, or curry powder with beef or lamb; rosemary or savory with chicken, fish, or veal. Season tomatoes with curry powder, basil, or oregano; turnips with rosemary; cabbage with savory; zucchini or carrots with thyme or nutmeg; cauliflower with dill; spinach with marjoram or nutmeg.

The addition of seasoning salt and lemon pepper to recipes gives an entirely new taste.

To enhance dishes, use a variety of condiments in lieu of salt: chervil for soups and eggs (½ teaspoon for 4 servings); Beau Monde for eggs, fish, meats, sauces, and stuffing (½ teaspoon for 4 servings). Mei Yen in shrimp soufflé (1½ teaspoons) or 1 tablespoon to either 4 eggs or 3 cups milk in other soufflés. Bay leaf, celery salt, or marjoram (1 teaspoon to 1 teaspoon salt) for stews. Green onion seasoning (1 teaspoon to 4- to 6-pound chicken). Tarragon (2 teaspoons to 4- to 6-pound chicken) for stuffing. (Note: Beau Monde and Mei Yen are salt substitute condiments which contain traces of salt and sugar, and should, therefore, be used sparingly.)

Add herbs and spices to liquids. Ensure you thoroughly crush any whole spice or leaves—such as anise seed, basil, bay leaf, oregano, rosemary, thyme—or if left whole—such as bay leaf or cinnamon stick—remove before serving.

Interesting meals may be prepared if you are careful in selecting from your Exchange Lists. For instance, you may prepare a stew if you select one small potato from the Starch Exchange (List 4) and add vegetables and meat according to your own meal plan; or you might wish to have a spaghetti dinner by using spaghetti from the Starch Exchange (List 4), cheese from the Meat Exchange (List 5), and meat sauce.

Soy margarine and Soyamaise are good substitutes for margarine or butter; both have less fat content (if you are able to tolerate soy derivatives).

Use nondairy whips. Each cup averages about 160 calories. Note: Watch for coconut and palm oils, because coconut and palm oils are saturated fats.

Good sauces may be made from commercial sweet-and-sour barbecue sauce or teriyaki barbecue marinade—but be sure to check the sugar content.

Low-calorie diet spreads are available and may be used for sandwiches, hors d'oeuvres, and so on.

Unusual low-calorie or water-packed fruits, such as bing cherries, fruits for salads, Kadota figs, mandarin oranges, pineapple spears, and purple plums, are also available.

ADDITIONAL SUGGESTIONS

Measure dry ingredients before liquids; this will save washing utensils!

Sift flour *before* you measure when the recipe calls for sifted flour. Sift the flour into a bowl or onto a sheet of waxed paper, then spoon into measuring utensil. Level with a spatula or knife.

Molasses or syrup flows more easily if measuring utensil is rinsed in cold water and then lightly greased.

1 medium egg = ¼ cup eggs.

Have eggs at room temperature.

Arrowroot: 1 tablespoon = 1 Starch Exchange. (May be used to thicken fruit juice so juice can be used as spread.) Arrowroot powder may be used in place of flour; use half as much arrowroot as flour. In recipes which use arrowroot, flour may also be used, but be sure to double the amount.

Cornstarch: 2 tablespoons = 1 Starch Exchange. May be used to thicken fruit juice for use as spread.

Egg Yolk: 1 egg yolk = 1 Fat Exchange. Use in place of 1 tablespoon flour for thickening liquids. (Yields 3 grams protein, 5 grams fat, 300 grams cholesterol, and no carbohydrate. Note: Egg yolks are of different food value than flour and are high in cholesterol.)

Flour (all-purpose, sifted): 1 tablespoon = ⅓ Starch Exchange. 3 tablespoons = 1 Starch Exchange.

Tapioca: 1 teaspoon, no Exchange necessary. (This is used mostly for sweet sauces. In thickening power this is equivalent to 1 tablespoon flour.)

The following items are on the market and readily available:

Nondairy whipped topping (D-Zerta,
    Dream Whip)....................................1 tablespoon = 8 calories
    (can be found on the dessert shelf)

Nondairy whipped topping
    (Cool Whip)....................................1 tablespoon = 14 calories
    (can be found in the frozen food section)

Diet gelatin (D-Zerta) ....½ cup = 8 calories
    (can be found on the dessert shelf)

Diet margarine (Imperial, Weight
    Watchers)...1 tablespoon = 50 calories
    (can be found in the refrigerator section)

Sour half-and-half*...1 cup = 160 calories
    (can sometimes be found in refrigerator section)

Imitation sour cream (Imo)............................1 cup = 304 calories
(Note: This contains saturated fat, coconut and/or palm oil, and
therefore should be used sparingly.)

* Sour half-and-half can also be made using 1 cup half-and-half and 1 tablespoon
vinegar or lemon juice.

EATING OUT

The question most frequently asked by people on diabetic diets is "How do I make this diet fit my normal, daily routine?" This is extremely important both to children and adults. Size of portions will depend on individual calorie requirements and allowed food exchanges.

LUNCH-BOX MEALS
1. Starch Exchange: use either bread or crackers.
2. Fat Exchange: butter or mayonnaise; cream for beverages.
3. Fruit Exchange: use fresh fruit, unsweetened canned fruits, or fruit juices.
4. Meat Exchange: hard-boiled eggs, cold cuts, roast beef, turkey, chicken, ham, cheese, cottage cheese, peanut butter.
5. Milk Exchange: as beverage.
6. Vegetable Exchange: raw vegetables such as carrots, celery, cherry tomatoes, cucumber sticks, green pepper rings, radishes, whole tomatoes.

LUNCH-BOX SUGGESTIONS
SANDWICH: Composed of Starch Exchange (1 or 2 slices of bread), Meat Exchange (turkey or beef), Fat Exchange (butter or mayonnaise), and lettuce, sliced tomato, or other vegetable.

SANDWICH FILLINGS: for people on high-calorie diets, use chicken, egg, or tuna salad, for example.

SNACKS: graham crackers and butter
cheese and crackers

peanut butter and crackers
crackers and cold cuts, fish, or poultry

Examples

Milk (thermos or purchased at school)
Sandwich of turkey or peanut butter
Fresh fruit—apple or tangerine
Carrot and celery sticks

Sandwich or cheese and crackers or cottage cheese
Fresh fruit—pear
Fresh tomato
Coffee with cream or milk
Yogurt

HOT LUNCH PROGRAMS

Straight meat entrée with vegetables or plain hamburger sandwich or plain hot dog on a bun
Fresh fruit
Salad with controlled diet dressing
Beverage—water, milk, coffee, or tea

Assortment from List 2: raw vegetable as desired, without sauces
Cold baked chicken
Bread and butter
Fresh fruit
Milk or hot beverage, as desired

DINING OUT HINTS

It can be easy to dine out comfortably on your calorie-restricted diet if you keep your exchange groupings in mind. Avoid dishes you are unsure of, such as casseroles, creamed foods, and other dishes that might have "hidden" ingredients.

1. Order plain soups, such as consommé, French onion, vegetable.
2. When ordering a salad, ask for your dressing "on the side" so you can measure the amount according to the fat exchanges you are allowed for that meal. If your fat exchanges are limited, a lemon wedge or vinegar (wine or cider) is usually available upon request.

Sliced tomatoes are usually available upon request. Order them without dressing or with the dressing on the side.

3. In selecting entrées, choose meat items that are either baked, broiled, poached, or roasted. Ask the restaurant to eliminate butter from their preparation. The following are recommended:

   a. Baked or broiled chicken.
   b. Broiled shish-kabob or brochette without marinade.
   c. Broiled or baked seafood or fish.
   d. Broiled steak.
   e. Hamburger steak.
   f. Prime rib, roast beef.
   g. Roast turkey (account for dressing and gravy in appropriate food groups).

   Request that sauces and gravies be eliminated from your entrée or brought separately.

4. Order hot and cold cereals plain. Use milk or cream on cereals according to your exchange pattern.
5. Order bread or rolls without fat, according to your exchange pattern. Order toast dry.
6. Plain potatoes are readily available, either baked or boiled. For oven-browned or mashed potato, figure one Starch Exchange plus one Fat Exchange.
7. Order cooked vegetables plain; if not available, figure one extra Fat Exchange per serving of vegetables.
8. Recommended vegetables commonly served in restaurants include green beans, tomatoes, carrots, peas, corn on the cob, mixed vegetables, asparagus.
9. Order eggs poached or soft cooked; for fried or scrambled eggs, if prepared in a skillet, add one Fat Exchange.
10. Order bacon or sausage crisp.*

---

* Nonetheless, these are still fats and should be considered as such.

11. Fresh fruit is usually available (in season); choose banana, half grapefruit (plain), melon wedge, or fresh strawberries. Stewed prunes are often available without sugar syrup.
12. Order unsweetened fruit juice, or fresh fruit juice.
13. Order yogurt (plain) in lieu of sour cream.

DAILY MENU GUIDE

Eat your meals at about the same time every day. Eat only the amounts given on your diet plan and do not skip meals.

Use of the exchange lists is based on the recommendations of the American Diabetes Association and The American Dietetic Association in cooperation with the National Institute of Arthritis, Metabolism, and Digestive Diseases, and the National Heart and Lung Institute of the U.S. Public Health Service, Department of Health and Human Services.

Since an adequate understanding of this diet is essential to its proper use, consultation with a professional (preferably a physician, dietition, or nurse) is recommended at the time you are given the diet and at regular intervals as needed. For additional information regarding "Exchange Lists for Meal Planning" contact your local American Diabetes Association Affiliate, listed in the white pages of your phone book, or write the American Diabetes Association, National Service Center, Order Department at 1660 Duke Street, Alexandria, VA 22314.

INSTRUCTIONS FOR DAILY MENU GUIDE

The foods allowed in your diet should be selected from the exchange lists. Menus should be planned on the basis of the daily menu guide. Foods in the same list are interchangeable because, in the quantities specified, they provide approximately the same amounts of carbohydrate, protein, and fat. For example, when our menu calls for one Starch Exchange, any item in List 4 may be used in the amount stated. If two Starch Exchanges are allowed, double the specified amount of one item or use one Exchange of each of *two* foods in List 4. A day's sample menus are given to illustrate correct use of the exchange lists.

CALORIE DIETS

The following suggested diets include a breakdown of exchange lists for breakfast, lunch, and dinner.

1000 Calories (approximately)

carbohydrate..... 130 gm
protein........... 55 gm
fat............... 30 gm

Breakfast	Breakfast (Example)
1½ Fruit Exchanges (List 3)	Orange juice........... ¾ cup
2 Starch Exchanges (List 4)	Toast .... 1 slice
	Cereal, dry .... ¾ cup
1 Fat Exchange (List 6)	Margarine .... 1 tsp.
½ cup nonfat milk (List 1)	Nonfat milk .... ½ cup

Lunch	Lunch (Example)
2 Meat Exchanges (List 5)	Cheese........ two 1-oz. slices
1 Starch Exchange (List 4)	Bread................. 1 slice
Vegetable(s) as desired (List 2)	Dill pickles, radishes as desired
1 Fruit Exchange (List 3)	Apple................ 1 small
½ cup nonfat milk (List 1)	Nonfat milk .... ½ cup
	Mustard .... as desired

Dinner	Dinner (Example)
2 Meat Exchanges (List 5)	Chicken, baked .... 2 oz.
1 Starch Exchange (List 4)	Peas .... ½ cup
1 Vegetable Exchange (List 2)	Tomatoes .... ½ cup
Vegetable(s) as desired (List 2)	Lettuce, endive ..... as desired
1½ Fruit Exchanges (List 3)	Fruit cocktail .... ¾ cup
1 Fat Exchange (List 6)	Margarine .... 1 tsp.
½ cup nonfat milk (List 1)	Nonfat milk .... ½ cup

Bedtime Feeding	Bedtime Feeding (Example)
½ Starch Exchange (List 4)	Graham cracker ... 1½ squares
½ cup nonfat milk (List 1)	Nonfat milk .... ½ cup

1200 Calories (approximately)

carbohydrate..... 145 gm
protein........... 55 gm
fat............... 30 gm

Breakfast	*Breakfast (Example)*
1½ Fruit Exchanges (List 3)	Orange juice........... ¾ cup
1 Starch Exchange (List 4)	Toast .... 1 slice
1 Meat Exchange (List 5)	Egg....................... 1
1 Fat Exchange (List 6)	Margarine .... 1 tsp.
1 cup nonfat milk (List 1)	Nonfat milk........... 1 cup

Lunch	*Lunch (Example)*
2 Meat Exchanges (List 5)	Cheese .... two 1-oz. slices
	Beef bouillon .... as desired
2 Starch Exchanges (List 4)	Bread................. 1 slice
	Saltine crackers 6
1 Vegetable Exchange (List 2)	Carrot and celery
	sticks................ ½ cup
1 Fruit Exchange (List 3)	Apple................ 1 small
1 Fat Exchange (List 6)	Margarine .... 1 tsp.
½ cup nonfat milk (List 1)	Nonfat milk .... ½ cup
	Mustard .... as desired

Dinner	*Dinner (Example)*
2 Meat Exchanges (List 5)	Chicken, baked .... 2 oz.
1 Starch Exchange (List 4)	Potatoes, mashed....... ½ cup
1 Vegetable Exchange (List 2)	Tomatoes .... ½ cup
Vegetable(s) as desired (List 2)	Lettuce, radishes .... as desired
1 Fruit Exchange (List 3)	Fruit cocktail .... ½ cup
1 Fat Exchange (List 6)	Margarine .... 1 tsp.

Bedtime Feeding	*Bedtime Feeding (Example)*
1 Starch Exchange (List 4)	Graham crackers .... 3 squares
½ cup nonfat milk (List 1)	Nonfat milk .... ½ cup

1500 Calories (approximately)   carbohydrate . . . . . 195 gm
protein . . . . 75 gm
fat . . . . 50 gm

Breakfast
2 Fruit Exchanges (List 3)
2 Starch Exchanges (List 4)

1 Meat Exchange (List 5)
1 Fat Exchange (List 6)
1 cup nonfat milk (List 1)

Breakfast (Example)
Orange juice . . . . 1 cup
Cereal, dry . . . . ¾ cup
Toast . . . . 1 slice
Egg. 1
Margarine . . . . 1 tsp.
Nonfat milk. . . . . 1 cup

Lunch
3 Meat Exchanges (List 5)
2 Starch Exchanges (List 4)
1 Vegetable Exchange (List 2)

2 Fruit Exchanges (List 3)
1 Fat Exchange (List 6)

Lunch (Example)
Cheese . . . . three 1-oz. slices
Bread . . . . 2 slices
Carrot and celery
    sticks . . . . ½ cup
Apples . . . . 2 small
Mayonnaise-type dressing 2 tsp.

Dinner
3 Meat Exchanges (List 5)
2 Starch Exchanges (List 4)

2 Vegetable Exchanges (List 2)
Vegetable(s) as desired (List 2)
1 Fruit Exchange (List 3)
1 Fat Exchange (List 6)
½ cup nonfat milk (List 1)

Dinner (Example)
Chicken, baked . . . . 3 oz.
Peas . . . . ½ cup
Potatoes, mashed . . . . ½ cup
Tomatoes . . . . 1 cup
Lettuce, chicory . . . . . as desired
Fruit cocktail . . . . ½ cup
Margarine . . . . 1 tsp.
Nonfat milk . . . . ½ cup
Salad dressing,
    fat-free . . . . 1 Tbsp.

Bedtime Feeding
1 Starch Exchange (List 4)
½ cup nonfat milk (List 1)

Bedtime Feeding (Example)
Graham crackers . . . . 3 squares
Nonfat milk . . . . ½ cup

1800 Calories (approximately)   carbohydrate. . . . . 225 gm
                                      protein. . . . . 90 gm
                                      fat. . . . . 60 gm

Breakfast   *Breakfast (Example)*
2 Fruit Exchanges (List 3)   Orange juice . . . . 1 cup
2 Starch Exchanges (List 4)   Toast . . . . 2 slices
1 Meat Exchange (List 5)   Egg. 1
1 Fat Exchange (List 6)   Margarine . . . . 1 tsp.
1 cup nonfat milk (List 1)   Nonfat milk. . . . . 1 cup

Lunch   *Lunch (Example)*
2 Meat Exchanges (List 5)   Cold cuts . . . . . . two 1-oz. slices
                               Cheese . . . . 1 oz.
2 Starch Exchanges (List 4)   Bread . . . . 2 slices
1 Vegetable Exchange (List 2) Carrot and celery
                                  sticks. . . . . ½ cup
2 Fruit Exchanges (List 3)   Banana . . . . 1 small
                               Apple. . . . . 1 small
2 Fat Exchanges (List 6)   Mayonnaise-type
                                  dressing . . . . 4 tsp.

Dinner   *Dinner (Example)*
3 Meat Exchanges (List 5)   Chicken, baked . . . . 3 oz.
3 Starch Exchanges (List 4)   Peas . . . . ½ cup
                               Potatoes, mashed. . . . . . . ½ cup
                               Bread. . . . . 1 slice
2 Vegetable Exchanges (List 2) Tomatoes . . . . 1 cup
Vegetable(s) as desired (List 2) Lettuce, escarole . . . . as desired
1 Fruit Exchange (List 3)   Fruit cocktail . . . . ½ cup
2 Fat Exchanges (List 6)   Margarine . . . . 2 tsp.
½ cup nonfat milk (List 1)   Nonfat milk . . . . ½ cup
                               (Salad dressing,
                                  fat-free) . . . . 1 Tbsp.

Bedtime Feeding
2 Starch Exchanges (List 4)
1 Meat Exchange (List 5)
½ cup nonfat milk (List 1)

Bedtime Feeding (Example)
Bread . . . . 2 slices
Roast beef, lean . . . . 1 oz.
Nonfat milk . . . . ½ cup
Mustard . . . . as desired

2000 Calories (approximately)
carbohydrate. . . . . 245 gm
protein. . . . . 110 gm
fat. . . . . 65 gm

Breakfast
2 Fruit Exchanges (List 3)
2 Starch Exchanges (List 4)

1 Meat Exchange (List 5)
2 Fat Exchanges (List 6)

1 cup nonfat milk (List 1)

Breakfast (Example)
Orange juice . . . . 1 cup
Cereal, dry . . . . ¾ cup
Toast . . . . 1 slice
Egg. 1
Bacon, crisp . . . . 1 slice
Margarine . . . . 1 tsp.
Nonfat milk. . . . . 1 cup

Lunch
3 Meat Exchanges (List 5)

2 Starch Exchanges (List 4)
Vegetable(s) as desired (List 2)

1 Vegetable Exchange (List 2)

2 Fruit Exchanges (List 3)
1 Fat Exchange (List 6)

1 cup nonfat milk (List 1)

Lunch (Example)
Cold cuts . . . . . two 1-oz. slices
Cheese . . . . 1 oz.
Bread . . . . 2 slices
Dill pickles,
    radishes . . . . as desired
Carrot and celery
    sticks. . . . . ½ cup
Apples . . . . 2 small
Mayonnaise-type
    dressing . . . . 2 tsp.
Nonfat milk. . . . . 1 cup

Dinner	*Dinner (Example)*
3 Meat Exchanges (List 5)	Chicken, baked . . . . 3 oz.
3 Starch Exchanges (List 4)	Peas . . . . ½ cup
	Potatoes, mashed . . . . ½ cup
	Bread . . . . 1 slice
2 Vegetable Exchanges (List 2)	Tomatoes . . . . 1 cup
Vegetable(s) as desired (List 2)	Lettuce, etc. . . . . as desired
1 Fruit Exchange (List 3)	Fruit cocktail . . . . ½ cup
1 Fat Exchange (List 6)	Margarine . . . . 1 tsp.
1 cup nonfat milk (List 1)	Nonfat milk . . . . 1 cup
	Salad dressing, fat-free . . . . 1 Tbsp.

Bedtime Feeding	*Bedtime Feeding (Example)*
2 Starch Exchanges (List 4)	Bread . . . . 2 slices
2 Meat Exchanges (List 5)	Roast beef, lean . . . . 2 oz.
1 Fruit Exchange (List 3)	Grapes 17
	Mustard . . . . as desired

2500 Calories (approximately)

carbohydrate . . . . . 315 gm
protein . . . . 120 gm
fat . . . . 85 gm

Breakfast	*Breakfast (Example)*
2 Fruit Exchanges (List 3)	Orange juice . . . . 1 cup
3 Starch Exchanges (List 4)	Cereal, dry . . . . ¾ cup
	Toast . . . . 2 slices
1 Meat Exchange (List 5)	Egg 1
2 Fat Exchanges (List 6)	Margarine . . . . 2 tsp.
1 cup nonfat milk (List 1)	Nonfat milk . . . . 1 cup

Midmorning Feeding	*Midmorning Feeding (Example)*
1 Starch Exchange (List 4)	Graham crackers . . . . 3 squares
½ cup nonfat milk (List 1)	Nonfat milk . . . . ½ cup

Lunch	**Lunch (Example)**
2 Meat Exchanges (List 5)	Triple-decker sandwich:
	Cold cuts .... two 1-oz. slices
	Cheese................ 1 oz.
3 Starch Exchanges (List 4)	Bread.............. 3 slices
3 Fat Exchanges (List 6)	Mayonnaise-type
	dressing............. 2 tsp.
	Margarine .... 2 tsp.
2 Vegetable Exchanges (List 2)	Carrot and celery
	sticks .... 1 cup
1 Fruit Exchange (List 3)	Apple................ 1 small
1 cup nonfat milk (List 1)	Nonfat milk........... 1 cup

Midafternoon Feeding	**Midafternoon Feeding (Example)**
1 Starch Exchange (List 4)	Saltine crackers 6
1 Fruit Exchange (List 3)	Pineapple juice......... ½ cup

Dinner	**Dinner (Example)**
3 Meat Exchanges (List 5)	Chicken, baked .... 3 oz.
3 Starch Exchanges (List 4)	Peas .... ½ cup
	Potatoes, mashed....... ½ cup
	Bread................ 1 slice
2 Vegetable Exchanges (List 2)	Tomatoes .... 1 cup
Vegetable(s) as desired (List 2)	Lettuce, radishes .... as desired
1 Fruit Exchange (List 3)	Fruit cocktail .... ½ cup
3 Fat Exchanges (List 6)	Margarine .... 3 tsp.
1 cup nonfat milk (List 1)	Nonfat milk........... 1 cup

Bedtime Feeding	**Bedtime Feeding (Example)**
2 Starch Exchanges (List 4)	Hamburger bun........... 1
2 Meat Exchanges (List 5)	Roast beef, lean .... 2 oz.
1 Fat Exchange (List 6)	Mayonnaise-type
	dressing .... 2 tsp.
½ cup nonfat milk (List 1)	Nonfat milk........... ½ cup

3000 Calories (approximately)   carbohydrate..... 300 gm
protein.......... 140 gm
fat.............. 135 gm

Breakfast	*Breakfast (Example)*
1 Fruit Exchange (List 3)	Orange juice........... ½ cup
3 Starch Exchanges (List 4)	Cereal, dry .... ¾ cup
	Toast .... 2 slices
2 Meat Exchanges (List 5)	Eggs....................... 2
4 Fat Exchanges (List 6)	Bacon, crisp........... 2 slices
	Margarine .... 2 tsp.
1 cup 2% fat milk (List 1)	Milk, 2% fat............ 1 cup

Midmorning Feeding	*Midmorning Feeding (Example)*
1 cup 2% fat milk (List 1)	Milk, 2% fat............ 1 cup
1 Starch Exchange (List 4)	Graham crackers.... 3 squares

Lunch	*Lunch (Example)*
3 Meat Exchanges (List 5)	Sandwich:
3 Starch Exchanges (List 4)	Cheese................ 1 oz.
3 Fat Exchanges (List 6)	Mayonnaise-type
	dressing............. 2 tsp.
	Bread .... 1 slice
	Sandwich:
	Cold cut ..... two 1-oz. slices
	Mayonnaise-type
	dressing............. 2 tsp.
	Margarine .... 1 tsp.
	Bread............... 2 slices
1 Vegetable Exchange (List 2)	Carrot and celery
	sticks................ ½ cup
1 Fruit Exchange (List 3)	Apple................ 1 small
1 cup 2% fat milk (List 1)	Milk, 2% fat............ 1 cup

Midafternoon Feeding

1 Meat Exchange (List 5)
2 Starch Exchanges (List 4)

Dinner

3 Meat Exchanges (List 5)
2½ Starch Exchanges (List 4)

1 Vegetable Exchange (List 2)
Vegetable(s) as desired (List 2)
1 Fruit Exchange (List 3)
1 cup 2% fat milk (List 1)
3 Fat Exchanges (List 6)

Bedtime Feeding

1 Meat Exchange (List 5)
2 Starch Exchanges (List 4)
2 Fat Exchanges (List 6)
1 cup 2% fat milk (List 1)

**Midafternoon Feeding
(Example)**

Frankfurter. 1
Frankfurter roll 1

Dinner (Example)

Chicken, baked . . . . 3 oz.
Peas . . . . ½ cup
Potatoes, mashed . . . . ½ cup
Bread . . . . ½ slice
Tomatoes . . . . ½ cup
Lettuce, escarole . . . . as desired
Fruit cocktail . . . . ½ cup
Milk, 2% fat. . . . . 1 cup
Margarine . . . . 3 tsp.

Bedtime Feeding (Example)

Roast beef, lean . . . . 1 oz.
Hamburger bun 1
Margarine . . . . 2 tsp.
Milk, 2% fat. . . . . 1 cup
Mustard . . . . as desired

APPETIZERS AND BEVERAGES

One serving is equivalent to 3½ ounces or 100 grams.

When using basic ingredients such as arrowroot, eggs, flour, margarine, and tapioca, refer to Weights, Measures, and the Metric System, Notes on Special Ingredients Used in Recipes, and Additional Suggestions (see Contents).

HONOLULU DIP

Exchanges per serving: ¼ cup = 2 Fat
Calories per serving: 90 (for dip only)   Yield: 1½ cups

½ cup chopped fresh (or crushed, artificially sweetened) pineapple
2 tablespoons chopped mint
3 ounces Neufchâtel cream cheese
2 tablespoons safflower mayonnaise

Blend ingredients together. Serve with crisp carrot and celery sticks and crackers.

GOLDEN SHOYU DIP

Exchanges per serving: 2 tablespoons = 2 Fat
Calories per serving: 90   Yield: 1¼ cups

1 cup safflower mayonnaise
¼ cup soy sauce
½ teaspoon instant onion
¼ teaspoon arrowroot

Blend all ingredients until smooth. Chill. Restir before serving as dip for all fish "pupus," or with grilled or fried fish.

CHEESE NIBBLERS

Exchanges per serving: 1 ball = ¼ Starch, ¼ Fat, ¼ Meat
Calories per serving: 40   Yield: 36 nibblers

½ cup sharp cheddar cheese, grated	½ cup diet margarine 1 cup flour

Mix ingredients together and roll into balls. (These can be made ahead of time and frozen.) To bake, place in a preheated 375°F oven for 15 minutes. If frozen, bake for 20–25 minutes.

CHEESE AND PINEAPPLE PUPUS

Exchanges per serving: ⅓ cup dip = 3 Fat, ¾ High-Fat Meat
                          ½ cup pineapple = ¾ fruit
Calories per serving: 250   Yield: Fruit, 4 cups
                                              Sauce, 3 cups

1 whole fresh pineapple, cubed*	1 cup cheddar cheese, grated
1½ cups diet mayonnaise	½ cup shredded unsweetened coconut

Serve pineapple chunks on picks with other ingredients in bowls. Dip pineapple first in mayonnaise, then in cheese and coconut.

* 1 average pineapple makes approximately 4 cups.

RUMAKI

Exchanges per serving: 4 rumakis = 1 Meat
Calories per serving: 125   Yield: 48 rumakis

12 chicken livers	1 cup water chestnuts,
1 teaspoon seasoned salt	drained
⅛ teaspoon ginger	16 slices bacon

Cut livers into small bite-size pieces and season with salt and
ginger; cut water chestnuts into halves and bacon into thirds.
Wrap each piece of liver with a half chestnut in bacon and secure with a pick. Broil or bake in 425°F oven until golden
brown (25–30 minutes). Serve with hot fruit chutney, chili
sauce, Chinese mustard, or Hot Shoyu Sauce (see Index).

YUMMY COFFEE DRINK

Exchanges per serving: 1 cup = 1 Fat
Calories per serving: 45   Yield: 4½ cups

2 cups strong iced coffee	1 cup nondairy whipped
Nonnutritive sweetener	topping
equivalent to ⅓ cup	2 cups artificially
sugar	sweetened ginger ale

Mix coffee and sweetener. Fill 4 large glasses about ¼ full with
crushed ice. Add ¼ cup nondairy whipped topping to each
glass, ¼ cup coffee mixture, then ½ cup ginger ale. Stir slightly.

APPLE FOAM

Exchanges per serving: ⅓ cup = ¾ Fruit
Calories per serving: 40   Yield: 2 cups

2 cups apple juice	Dash of cinnamon
1 teaspoon lemon juice	¼ cup egg whites
Nonnutritive granulated	
sweetener equivalent to	
1½ cups sugar (reserve ½	
teaspoon)	

Chill juices. Mix ½ teaspoon reserved sweetener with cinnamon; set aside. Beat egg whites until stiff; add balance of sweetener while beating. Add apple and lemon juice; pour into fruit cups. Sprinkle with the cinnamon-sweetener mixture.

COCOA

Exchanges per serving: 1 cup = ¾ Skim Milk
Calories per serving: 70   Yield: 8 cups

6 tablespoons unsweetened cocoa	6 cups nonfat milk
½ teaspoon salt	Nonnutritive sweetener equivalent to ½ cup
2 cups water	sugar

Mix cocoa, salt, and water. Stir constantly over very low heat for 2 minutes. Add milk and sweetener; continue stirring until cocoa comes to a boil. Serve.

HOT CHOCOLATE

Exchanges per serving: ½ cup = 1 Fat, ½ Skim Milk
Calories per serving: 90   Yield: 2½ cups

1½ ounces unsweetened chocolate	Nonnutritive sweetener equivalent to ½ cup
¾ cup water	sugar
Dash of salt	2½ cups nonfat milk

Combine chocolate and water; cook, stirring constantly, until chocolate is melted. Add salt and sweetener; bring to boiling point; boil 4 minutes, stirring constantly. Place over boiling water, and gradually add milk, stirring constantly; heat. Just before serving, beat with rotary beater until frothy.

QUICK DRINK

Exchanges per serving: 1 cup = ½ Fruit, 1 Skim Milk
Calories per serving: 100   Yield: 1¼ cups

⅔ cup dry nonfat instant powdered milk
½ cup frozen fruit, unsweetened, or ½ cup fresh fruit
Nonnutritive sweetener equivalent to 2 tablespoons sugar
2 ice cubes
2 tablespoons water

Blend all ingredients in blender until ice cubes are dissolved.

JOAN'S FRUIT SHAKE

Exchanges per serving: 1 cup = ½ Fruit, ½ Skim Milk
Calories per serving: 80   Yield: 4 cups

2 bananas
3 tablespoons fresh orange juice
Dash of salt
Nonnutritive sweetener equivalent to ½ cup sugar
⅛ teaspoon vanilla
2 cups nonfat milk

Blend ingredients until smooth and foamy. Place in refrigerator until chilled, then blend again. Serve.

CRANBERRY PUNCH

Exchanges per serving: ½ cup = 1 Fruit
Calories per serving: 40   Yield: 15 cups

8 cups artificially sweetened cranberry juice cocktail
3 cups unsweetened pineapple juice
Nonnutritive sweetener equivalent to ½ cup sugar
4 cups artificially sweetened ginger ale

Combine juices and sweetener; chill. Stir in chilled ginger ale just before serving. Add ice cubes.

CRANBERRY SIP

Exchanges per serving: ½ cup = ¾ Fruit
Calories per serving: 30   Yield: 2½ cups

1 cup cranberries, washed
2 whole cloves
1 teaspoon cinnamon
1 cup water
Nonnutritive sweetener
  equivalent to 1½ cups
  sugar

¼ cup orange juice
¼ cup lemon juice
Dash of salt

Combine cranberries, spices, water, and sweetener; cook until cranberry skins burst. Strain; add remaining ingredients. Chill.

NONNIE'S CRANBERRY COCKTAIL

Exchanges per serving: ½ cup = ¾ Fruit
Calories per serving: 40   Yield: 5 cups

4 cups artificially
  sweetened cranberry
  juice
3 cloves
1 stick cinnamon

Nonnutritive sweetener
  equivalent to 1 cup sugar
¼ cup fresh lemon juice
⅔ cup fresh orange juice
Dash of salt

Combine first four ingredients; bring to a boil. Reduce heat; simmer a few minutes, then remove from heat. Add citrus juices and salt; chill. Serve very cold.

APRICOT ORANGE PUNCH

Exchanges per serving: ½ cup = 1 Fruit
Calories per serving: 60   Yield: 7 cups

1½ cups artificially
sweetened apricot nectar
3 cups fresh orange juice
½ cup fresh lemon juice

Nonnutritive sweetener
equivalent to ½ cup
sugar
2 cups artificially
sweetened ginger ale

Combine first four ingredients; chill well. Just before placing in
punch bowl, add well-chilled ginger ale.

COFFEE PUNCH

Exchanges per serving: 1 cup = 1 Skim Milk
Calories per serving: 80   Yield: 24 6-ounce cups

2 cups nonfat milk
8 cups strong coffee, cold
2 teaspoons vanilla
Nonnutritive sweetener
equivalent to ½ cup
sugar

4 cups ice milk (vanilla,
chocolate, or coffee)
1 cup nondairy whipped
topping
Dash of cinnamon or
nutmeg

Combine milk, coffee, vanilla, and sweetener in large pitcher;
stir until sweetener dissolves; chill. Place chunks of ice milk in
punch bowl just before serving. Add coffee mix, top with
nondairy whipped topping, stir lightly; sprinkle with cinnamon
or nutmeg.

"DELISHUS" PUNCH

Exchanges per serving: ½ cup = ½ Fruit
Calories per serving: 40   Yield: 8 cups

1 dozen cloves, whole
1 orange, thinly sliced
1 lemon, thinly sliced
4 cups artificially
   sweetened cranberry
   juice cocktail

1 cinnamon stick
1 teaspoon allspice
2 tablespoons lemon juice
Nonnutritive sweetener to
   taste

Put a clove in each slice of orange and lemon. Place fruit slices
in a pitcher. Combine cranberry cocktail and spices; heat to boiling over low heat. Add lemon juice; add sweetener to taste and
strain hot mixture into pitcher over fruit. Serve in punch cups
garnished with fruit slices.

OLGA'S MINTY DRINK

Exchanges per serving: 1 cup = ½ Fruit
Calories per serving: 40   Yield: 8 cups

¼ cup mint leaves,
   chopped fine
Nonnutritive sweetener
   equivalent to ½ cup
   sugar

1 cup water
½ cup fresh lemon juice
2 cups fresh orange juice
4 cups artificially
   sweetened ginger ale

Combine first three ingredients; bring to a boil. Cool and strain.
When ready to serve, add remaining ingredients; pour over
crushed ice in chilled glasses.

COLA DRINK

Exchanges per serving: 1 cup = ½ Skim Milk
Calories per serving: 80   Yield: 2 cups

2 teaspoons sugar-free,   Nonnutritive sweetener
   noncaloric cola   equivalent to 1 teaspoon
2 cups skim milk   sugar

Mix all ingredients well.

LEMONADE

Exchanges per serving: ½ cup = ½ Fruit
Calories per serving: 30   Yield: 2 cups

⅔ cup unsweetened lemon   Nonnutritive sweetener to
   juice   taste
1½ cups cold water   Lemon slices

Combine lemon juice and water. Sweeten with nonnutritive
sweetener. Pour into large glasses over ice. Garnish with lemon
slice.

LOU'S LEMONADE

Exchanges per serving: ½ cup = ¼ Fruit
Calories per serving: 20   Yield: 8 cups

1 cup unsweetened lemon   6 cups water
   juice   1 cup artificially sweetened
Nonnutritive sweetener   cranberry juice cocktail
   equivalent to ¾ cup
   sugar

Combine ingredients; mix well. Add ice cubes just prior to
serving.

EGGNOG DIVINE
(Not for diabetics without consent of doctor)

Exchanges per serving: ½ cup = ¼ Meat, ¾ Nonfat Milk
Calories per serving: 120   Yield: 5¼ cups
(alcohol is approximately 20)

3 eggs, separated
4 cups nonfat milk

Nonnutritive sweetener
equivalent to ½ cup
sugar
½ cup rum

Beat egg yolks until thick and lemony. Combine all ingredients except egg whites. Beat whites until stiff; fold in carefully just before serving.

NONALCOHOLIC EGGNOG

Exchanges per serving: 1 cup = ⅓ Skim Milk, ½ Meat
Calories per serving: 62   Yield: 4 cups

2 eggs
½ cup dry nonfat instant
powdered milk
2⅔ cups water, ice cold

Nonnutritive sweetener
equivalent to 2
tablespoons sugar
3 teaspoons vanilla
1 teaspoon rum flavoring

Place all ingredients in blender; mix well. Pour into cups and serve.

IMITATION WINE

Exchanges per serving: ½ cup = ½ Fruit
Calories per serving: 30   Yield: 8 cups

2 cups unsweetened grape
  juice
Nonnutritive sweetener
  equivalent to ½ cup
  sugar

2 cups artificially
  sweetened fruit-flavored
  carbonated beverage,
  chilled
4 cups artificially
  sweetened ginger ale,
  chilled

Combine juice and sweetener; chill. Stir in carbonated fruit-flavored beverage and ginger ale just before serving. Add ice cubes.

WINE LEMONADE
(Not for diabetics without consent of doctor)

Exchanges per serving: 1 cup = None
Calories per serving: 260   Yield: 5½ cups
(alcohol is approximately 240)

3 cups water
½ cup fresh lemon juice

Nonnutritive sweetener
  equivalent to ½ cup
  sugar
2 cups white wine

Combine all ingredients; pour over crushed ice in chilled glasses.

SOUPS

JOAN'S JELLIED TOMATO CONSOMMÉ

Exchanges per serving: ⅔ cup = 1 Vegetable
Calories per serving: 45   Yield: 3 cups

1 envelope unflavored gelatin
2¼ cups tomato juice
1 bouillon cube, any flavor
½ teaspoon salt
Nonnutritive sweetener equivalent to ¼ cup sugar
½ teaspoon Worcestershire sauce
⅛ teaspoon Tabasco sauce
2 tablespoons lemon juice
¼ cup cucumbers, unpeeled and diced
½ cup sour half-and-half or low-fat plain yogurt (optional)

Sprinkle gelatin over half the tomato juice in a saucepan. Add bouillon cube; place over low heat, stirring constantly until gelatin and cube are dissolved (about 3 minutes). Remove from heat. Add rest of tomato juice, salt, sweetener, Worcestershire and Tabasco sauces, lemon juice, and cucumbers. Pour into 2″ × 8″ × 8″ pan; chill until firm. Spoon into serving dishes; serve with sour half-and-half or plain low-fat yogurt, if desired.

ASPARAGUS SOUP

Exchanges per serving: ½ cup = 1 Vegetable
Calories per serving: 12   Yield: 5 cups

2 cups asparagus, cooked
3 cups water
4 bouillon cubes, any flavor
Dash of thyme
⅛ teaspoon salt
Dash of pepper

Puree asparagus. Boil water; combine with bouillon cubes, thyme, salt, and pepper; add asparagus; simmer 5 minutes.

CUCUMBER SOUP

Exchanges per serving: 1 cup = 1 Vegetable
Calories per serving: 35   Yield: 4 cups

2 beef or chicken bouillon cubes
2 cups water
1½ cups cucumber, sliced
½ cup plain yogurt made from skim milk
¼ teaspoon lemon peel, dried
Dash of seasoned salt
Dash of pepper
Dash of thyme

Bring bouillon cubes, water, and cucumber slices to boil. Cover and simmer until cucumber is tender (about 10 minutes). Cool and place in refrigerator. When cold, blend; add yogurt, lemon peel, and seasonings. Blend until smooth. Serve cold.

VEGETABLE SOUP, COLD
(Gazpacho)

Exchanges per serving: ½ cup = 1 Vegetable
Calories per serving: 30   Yield: 5 cups

1 cup tomatoes, peeled and finely chopped
½ cup green pepper, finely chopped (remove core)
½ cup celery, finely chopped
½ cup cucumber, peeled and finely chopped
¼ cup green onion, finely chopped
2 teaspoons parsley, snipped
1 teaspoon chives, snipped
1 small clove garlic, minced (put through garlic press)
3 tablespoons tarragon wine vinegar
1 teaspoon garlic salt
¼ teaspoon pepper
1 teaspoon Worcestershire sauce
2 cups tomato juice
Tabasco sauce to taste (approximately 2 teaspoons)

Combine ingredients in either a glass or a stainless steel bowl. Put half the mixture through blender. When thoroughly blended, return to bowl; mix well. Cover bowl and place in refrigerator to chill at least 4 hours; serve in chilled cups. This may also be served in place of a salad.

GREAT CARROT (OR BEAN) SOUP

Exchanges per serving: 1 cup = ⅔ Vegetable
Calories per serving: 25   Yield: 3 cups

1 cup water	¼ teaspoon thyme
2 bouillon cubes, any flavor	Dash of salt
	Dash of pepper
2 scant cups carrots (or green beans, if preferred)	

Heat water with bouillon cubes in saucepan; stir occasionally. Add carrots; puree until smooth. Add thyme, salt, and pepper.

TARRAGON SOUP

Exchanges per serving: ⅔ cup = ¼ Fat, 1 Vegetable
Calories per serving: 40   Yield: 2⅓ cups

2 tablespoons onion, chopped	2 cups tomato juice
2 tablespoons celery, chopped very fine	½ teaspoon dried tarragon
	½ teaspoon salt
1 tablespoon diet margarine	⅛ teaspoon pepper
	Dash of Tabasco sauce, if desired

Sauté onion and celery in margarine until onion is golden; add remaining ingredients. Bring to a boil. Lower heat; simmer 5 minutes.

EASY PEANUT SOUP

Exchanges per serving: ⅔ cup = 1 Starch, ½ Fat
Calories per serving: 134   Yield: 4¾ cups

1½ cups cream of chicken   ¼ cup chunky peanut
 soup   butter
1½ cups cream of celery   1½ cups water
 soup

Blend all ingredients well; let simmer 5 minutes.

POTATO AND WATERCRESS SOUP

Exchanges per serving: 1 cup = ½ Starch, ½ Fat,
                               ½ Nonfat Milk
Calories per serving: 111   Yield: 3¼ cups

1⅓ cups cream of potato   ½ teaspoon thyme
 soup   Dash of salt
1⅓ cups nonfat milk   Dash of pepper
½ cup watercress, chopped
 fine (packed tightly)

Heat cream of potato soup with milk in saucepan. Puree watercress and thyme. Mix with soup until well blended. Add salt
and pepper. Cook 4 or 5 minutes over medium heat (or until
hot). Serve hot or cold.

CELERY BEAN SOUP

Exchanges per serving: 1 cup = ¼ Fat, ⅓ Skim Milk,
                               ⅓ Vegetable
Calories per serving: 70   Yield: 4 cups

1 cup string beans, cut fine   Dash of salt
2 tablespoons onion,   ⅔ teaspoon arrowroot
 chopped fine   powder
⅛ cup water   1½ cups nonfat milk
1¼ cups cream of celery
 soup

Combine beans and onion with water, soup, and tiny dash of salt. Cook in tightly covered saucepan about 6–7 minutes, until onions soften. In another saucepan combine a few grains of salt and arrowroot powder; stir in milk gradually to make a smooth mixture. Add to first mixture; cook over low heat, stirring occasionally until thickened. Adjust seasoning to taste.

FESTIVE TOMATO SOUP

Exchanges per serving: 1 scant cup = ½ Starch, ¾ Fruit
Calories per serving: 70   Yield: 5⅔ cups

2⅔ cups condensed tomato   ⅔ cup unsweetened
  soup   orange juice concentrate
                                              2½ cups water

Put tomato soup in pan; add mixture of orange juice and water. Boil gently. Serve hot or cold.

SHRIMP CHOWDER
(High cholesterol)

Exchanges per serving: 1 cup = ¼ Starch, 1½ Very Lean Meat,
                                                ¼ Skim Milk

Calories per serving: 130   Yield: 7½ cups

½ cup onion, finely
  chopped
1 tablespoon diet
  margarine
2 cups water
2 teaspoons salt
1¼ cups potatoes, pared
  and cubed (about ½"
  thick)

2 cups nonfat milk,
  scalded
12 ounces shrimp, drained
  and shelled (if shrimp are
  large, cut into smaller
  pieces)
½ tablespoon arrowroot
1 tablespoon water
Dash of pepper
Dash of salt

Sauté onion in margarine until golden. Add water, salt, and potatoes. Boil gently, covered, until potatoes are tender (about 20
minutes). Add scalded skim milk and shrimp, stirring occasionally. Bring to boil, reduce heat; simmer until shrimp are pink
and cooked (about 5 minutes). Make smooth thin paste of arrowroot and water; add to chowder and stir until slightly thickened. Add pepper and remaining salt, to taste.

SPLIT PEA SOUP

Exchanges per serving: 1 cup = ⅓ Starch, ⅓ Vegetable
Calories per serving: 40   Yield: 6 cups

1 cup green split peas
1 carrot, sliced thin
1 onion, sliced thin
5 cups water
3 beef or chicken bouillon
  cubes

1 teaspoon salt
Dash of pepper
1 teaspoon curry powder
  (optional)

Soak peas 2–3 hours in cold water, drain. Mix other ingredients
except curry powder together in a saucepan. Cover and boil

gently until peas are very soft (about 45 minutes). Stir in curry powder, if desired; press mixture through sieve and return puree to saucepan. Reheat and serve.

TURKEY-WATERCRESS SOUP

Exchanges per serving: 1 cup = 2 Lean Meat, ⅓ Vegetable
Calories per serving: 140   Yield: 3 cups

1 cup water	1½ cups cooked turkey,
1⅓ cups condensed turkey	cut in small pieces
broth	1 cup watercress, chopped
2 tablespoons onion,	fine (firmly packed)
chopped fine,	1½ teaspoons arrowroot
¼ cup celery, chopped fine	2 tablespoons water
½ teaspoon salt	

Simmer first six ingredients about 15 minutes. Add watercress and simmer again until watercress is wilted. Mix arrowroot and 2 tablespoons water into a smooth paste; stir into soup. Cook until clear and smooth (a few minutes).

QUICK AND TASTY CHICKEN SOUP

Exchanges per serving: 1 cup = 2 Lean Meat
Calories per serving: 140   Yield: 4 cups

1½ cups chicken, cooked	¼ cup celery, diced fine
and diced	½ teaspoon salt
1⅓ cups chicken broth	½ teaspoon thyme
1 cup water	½ tablespoon arrowroot
2 tablespoons onion,	1 tablespoon water
chopped fine	

Simmer first seven ingredients for about 10 minutes. Make paste of arrowroot and 1 tablespoon water, add to soup. Cook until clear and smooth (takes just a few seconds).

SALADS

NOTES

Many reduced calorie and "lite" salad dressings are now available in grocery stores. Look for products by Kraft, Wish-Bone, Light n' Lively, Roka, as well as others. Check the amount of calories per tablespoon, as it will vary by product, ranging from 7 to 50 calories per tablespoon.

Regular mayonnaise: 2 tablespoons = 200 calories
Mayonnaise whip: 2 tablespoons = 138 calories
Regular French dressing: 2 tablespoons = 150 calories
Diet French dressing: 2 tablespoons = 42 calories
(Note: Calories can be reduced by 5–15 calories with imitation mayonnaise or 25 calories with diet salad dressing.)

Vegetables that are so low in calories as to be unnecessary to count are celery, chicory, Chinese cabbage, endive, escarole, lettuce, parsley, peppers, radishes, and watercress.

SWEET AND SOUR CUCUMBER SALAD

Exchanges per serving: ½ cup = 1 Vegetable
Calories per serving: 20   Yield: 2 cups

½ cup water	2 tablespoons dill pickle,
1 cup cider vinegar	chopped fine
Nonnutritive sweetener	1½ teaspoons salt
equivalent to 2	2 cucumbers, sliced thin
tablespoons sugar	1 stalk celery, sliced thin

Boil water, vinegar, sweetener, pickle, and salt. Place cucumbers and celery slices in glass jar; pour boiling liquid over; cover and refrigerate overnight. Drain before serving.

MARINATED VEGETABLE TOSS

Exchanges per serving: ½ cup = 1 Vegetable
Calories per serving: 20 (excluding dressing)   Yield: 8 ½-cup
servings

2 cups fresh tomato   ½ cup celery crescents
  wedges, peeled   ½ cup cucumber chunks
½ cup radishes, sliced   Dietetic Italian dressing
½ medium red onion,
  thinly sliced

Combine all vegetables in salad bowl; pour Italian dressing
over. Refrigerate overnight.

RADISH CELERY SALAD

Exchanges per serving: ½ cup = 1 Vegetable
Calories per serving: 8   Yield: 2 cups

1 cup radishes, sliced thin   1 cup lettuce leaves,
1 cup celery, sliced thin   torn up
¼ cup French dressing
  (low-calorie)

Toss radishes, celery, and dressing together. Refrigerate an hour
or so before placing on lettuce leaves.

SWEET AND SOUR BEETS

Exchanges per serving: 1 serving = ½ Medium-Fat Meat,
                                         1½ Vegetable
Calories per serving: 77   Yield: 6 servings

4 cups sliced beets (reserve
juice)

Nonnutritive sweetener
equivalent to 3
tablespoons sugar

1 teaspoon salt

¼ teaspoon black pepper

1 tablespoon allspice

½ cup vinegar

3 eggs, hard-boiled and
shelled

2 cups lettuce, torn up

Mix ½ cup beet juice with sweetener, salt, pepper, and allspice.
Boil gently about 5 minutes. Strain; stir in vinegar. Place eggs
and beet slices in baking dish. Pour beet-juice mixture over; refrigerate overnight, turning both beets and eggs occasionally.
Slice eggs with egg slicer, drain beets and divide into 6 servings.
Place on lettuce leaves; top each with liquid; use half an egg for
each serving.

CARROT SLICES

Exchanges per serving: ⅔ cup = ½ Starch, 1 Vegetable, ¼ Fat
Calories per serving: 54   Yield: 3 cups

2 cups carrots, scraped and
cut into 1″ slices

¾ cup water

¼ cup cider vinegar

½ teaspoon dill pickle,
chopped fine

1 tablespoon green onion
seasoning

½ teaspoon poultry
seasoning

½ teaspoon thyme

¼ teaspoon garlic salt

½ teaspoon marjoram

½ teaspoon seasoned salt

Dash of lemon pepper

1 cup prepared croutons

Simmer first nine ingredients, covered, until carrots are tender.
Add salt, pepper, and croutons. Cool. Place in refrigerator for
an hour, drain, and serve.

MOTHER'S RAW SPINACH SALAD

Exchanges per serving: 1 cup = 2 Fat, 1 Vegetable
Calories per serving: 186   Yield: 5 servings

2 bunches fresh spinach
½ medium red onion,
  sliced thin and ringed
6 slices bacon, chopped
  and fried crisp

½ cup diet mayonnaise
½ cup wine vinegar
Nonnutritive sweetener
  equivalent to ½ cup
  sugar

Wash spinach thoroughly; cut off stems; crisp in refrigerator.
Tear into bite-size pieces in salad bowl; add onion rings and bacon bits. Combine mayonnaise, vinegar, and sweetener; mix
well in blender or mixer. Pour over greens. Toss and serve at
once.

HOT POTATO SALAD

Exchanges per serving: 1 cup = 1 Starch, 1 Lean Meat,
                                    1 Vegetable
Calories per serving: 138   Yield: 4 cups

2 cups potatoes, pared and
  cubed
Water
2½ teaspoons salt
1 onion, chopped fine
1 stalk celery, chopped fine

¼ cup green pepper,
  chopped fine
1 cup low-fat cottage
  cheese
2 cups lettuce leaves

Place potatoes in water to cover; cook until tender; drain. Toss
potato cubes and remaining ingredients together; mix well.
Serve on lettuce leaves.

TOMATO AND HERB SALAD

Exchanges per serving: 1 serving = 1 Vegetable
Calories per serving: 22   Yield: 6 servings

6 small tomatoes, peeled
1½ teaspoons oregano
Nonnutritive sweetener
    equivalent to 1
    tablespoon sugar

4 tablespoons malt vinegar
½ teaspoon seasoned salt
¼ teaspoon pepper
1 cup lettuce leaves,
    torn up

Chop 1½ tomatoes fine; combine with oregano, sweetener, vinegar, salt, and pepper. Slice remaining tomatoes, place on top of lettuce leaves; top with vinegar mix; refrigerate until ready to serve.

FROZEN ORANGE FRUIT SALAD

Exchanges per serving: ½ filled orange = 2½ Fat, 1 Fruit
Calories per serving: 199   Yield: 8 servings

4 oranges
¾ cup cream cheese*
½ cup diet mayonnaise or
    diet salad dressing
1 tablespoon lemon juice
¼ teaspoon prepared
    mustard
¼ teaspoon salt

1 cup unsweetened fruit
    cocktail, drained, or
    mixed unsweetened
    fruits
¼ cup slivered almonds
½ cup nondairy whipped
    topping sweetened to
    taste with artificial
    sweetener

Cut oranges in half and scoop out pulp. Combine cream cheese, mayonnaise, lemon juice, mustard, and salt. Add fruit cocktail, almonds, and drained orange pulp. Fold in whipped topping. Heap salad in orange halves; freeze until firm. Wrap individually in foil and keep frozen until needed. Remove from freezer ½ hour before serving. Garnish with endive or mint.

* See selections under Cheese and Egg Dishes.

PEPPER SLAW

Exchanges per serving: 1 cup = 1 Vegetable
Calories per serving: 26   Yield: 3 cups

½ head cabbage	¼ green pepper, chopped
2 cups water	fine
1 carrot, chopped fine	1 tablespoon mayonnaise-
	type dressing

Cut cabbage into small wedges. Place half in blender along with water, carrot, and pepper. Blend quickly; turn off and drain at once, using liquid for blending with balance of cabbage; drain once more. Mix with mayonnaise dressing.

CAESAR SALAD

Exchanges per serving: 1 cup = 2 Fat, ¾ Lean Meat,
                                      1 Vegetable
Calories per serving: 150   Yield: 6 servings

1 clove garlic	2-ounce can anchovy
1 head romaine lettuce or	fillets, drained and
1 head iceberg lettuce	chopped
¼ cup olive oil	¼ cup Parmesan cheese
Juice of 1 lemon	½ cup prepared croutons
¼ cup wine vinegar	1 egg, well beaten
	Salt and pepper to taste

Rub salad bowl with cut clove of garlic. Tear cleaned and crisped lettuce into bite-size pieces in salad bowl. Pour olive oil, lemon juice, and vinegar over greens; toss lightly. Sprinkle chopped anchovies, grated cheese, and croutons on top; add beaten egg. Season. Toss and serve at once.

JELLIED FRUIT SALAD

Exchanges per serving: ⅔ cup = ¾ Fruit
Calories per serving: 31   Yield: 4 cups

1 envelope low-calorie
   strawberry gelatin
   dessert
1¾ cups boiling water
¼ cup fresh lemon juice

Nonnutritive sweetener
   equivalent to ½ cup
   sugar
1 cup fresh peaches, sliced
   fine
1 cup cantaloupe balls

Dissolve gelatin in boiling water. Add lemon juice and sweetener. Chill until consistency of thick syrup; add fruits. Place in lightly oiled mold and chill until set.

MOLDED BEET-ONION SALAD

Exchanges per serving: ½ cup = 1 Vegetable
Calories per serving: 25   Yield: 4 servings

1 envelope black raspberry
   diet gelatin
2 cups boiling water

1 cup shoestring beets,
   drained
5-ounce jar cocktail
   pickled onions

Dissolve gelatin in boiling water. Chill until consistency of egg whites. Fold in vegetables. Pour in pan or molds; refrigerate until firm (5–6 hours).

PEACH-Y SALAD

Exchanges per serving: ⅔ cup = 1½ Fruit
Calories per serving: 69   Yield: 4 cups

4 cups artificially
   sweetened peaches,
   halved
1 tablespoon vinegar

2 sticks cinnamon
½ teaspoon allspice
1 teaspoon cloves, whole
2 cups torn lettuce leaves

Mix peaches, vinegar, cinnamon, and allspice. Boil gently 5 minutes. Place in refrigerator 5–6 hours. Drain thoroughly; stick a clove in each peach half; serve on lettuce.

ANN'S APPLE SALAD

Exchanges per serving: ½ cup = ½ Very Lean Meat, ¼ Fat, ¼ Fruit, ¼ Vegetable

Calories per serving: 70   Yield: 4 servings

½ cup apples, thinly sliced
½ cup low-fat cottage cheese
2 tablespoons diet salad dressing

½ cup carrots, grated
½ cup celery, chopped fine
Dash of salt
1 cup torn lettuce leaves

Toss together first six ingredients. Divide mixture and place about ½-cup portions on lettuce. Refrigerate before serving.

SUPER SALAD

Exchanges per serving: ⅔ cup = 1 Fruit, ½ Vegetable
Calories per serving: 58   Yield: 5 servings

1 cup carrots, grated
2 cups unsweetened pineapple tidbits (reserve syrup)
¼ teaspoon salt
½ teaspoon anise seed, crushed

1 tablespoon white vinegar
½ cup boiling water
⅛ cup lemon juice
1 envelope unflavored gelatin
2 cups torn lettuce leaves

Mix carrots, pineapple, salt, anise seed, vinegar, and water. Stir together lemon juice, gelatin, and syrup from pineapple; let soften; add to first mixture. Pour into lightly oiled salad mold. Refrigerate until firm. Loosen mold in hot water; run table knife along inside edges, invert on lettuce.

JELLIED APPLESAUCE SALAD

Exchanges per serving: ½ cup = 1 Fruit
Calories per serving: 54   Yield: 4 servings

1 envelope diet raspberry   ½ cup unsweetened
  gelatin   crushed pineapple,
1¾ cups boiling water   drained
1 cup unsweetened   ½ cup celery, chopped
  applesauce

Dissolve gelatin in hot water. Let cool in refrigerator until the
consistency of egg whites. Add fruits and celery; stir well. Pour
into pan or molds and refrigerate until set (4–5 hours).

APPLE-CELERY-CRANBERRY-NUT MOLD

Exchanges per serving: ¾ cup = 1½ Fat, 1 Fruit
Calories per serving: 101   Yield: 4¼ cups

2 cups cranberries   1 cup apples, peeled and
1¼ cups water   diced
Nonnutritive sweetener   ½ cup celery, chopped fine
  equivalent to 1 cup sugar   ½ cup pecans, chopped
1 envelope unflavored   very fine
  gelatin   Lettuce

Cook cranberries in 1 cup water. When skins are broken, rub
through sieve. Add sweetener and reheat. Soften gelatin in remaining ¼ cup water; add to cranberry puree; cool. When mixture starts to thicken, add apples, celery, and pecans. Pour into
mold. Chill. Serve on lettuce.

GOLDEN GLOW SALAD

Exchanges per serving: ½ cup = ½ Fruit, ½ Vegetable
Calories per serving: 37   Yield: 4 cups

1 envelope unflavored
gelatin
⅛ cup lemon juice
2 cups artificially
sweetened pineapple
tidbits (reserve juice)

¼ teaspoon salt
1 tablespoon vinegar
1 cup carrots, grated
½ cup boiling water
2 cups torn lettuce leaves

Mix gelatin, lemon juice, and juice from pineapple tidbits.
Soften gelatin a few minutes; stir in salt, vinegar, carrots,
pineapple, and boiling water. Pour into 9″ × 5″ × 3″ loaf pan; refrigerate until firm (about 4 hours). Serve on lettuce bed.

RASPBERRY RHUBARB SALAD

Exchanges per serving: ½ cup = ½ Vegetable
Calories per serving: 20 (excluding dressing)   Yield: 4 cups

1 envelope sugar-free
raspberry gelatin
1 cup boiling water
½ cup artificially
sweetened cooked
rhubarb

½ teaspoon anise seed,
crushed fine
½ cup apples, chopped fine
½ cup celery, chopped fine
1 or 2 drops red vegetable
coloring
2 cups lettuce, chopped

Dissolve gelatin and food coloring in water. Add rhubarb and
anise seed; mix well. Cool until congealed slightly. Add apples
and celery; mix well. Pour into slightly oiled 1 quart salad mold;
chill until firm. Divide equally on lettuce and serve with fruit
salad dressing, if desired.

MOLDED VEGETABLE SALAD

Exchanges per serving: ½ cup = ½ Vegetable
Calories per serving: 17   Yield: 4 servings

1 envelope diet orange
   gelatin
2 cups boiling water
½ cup white cabbage,
   chopped

½ cup carrots, shredded
¼ cup celery, finely
   chopped
¼ teaspoon celery seeds

Dissolve gelatin in boiling water. Chill until consistency of egg
white. Fold in vegetables and celery seeds. Pour in 1 quart mold
and refrigerate until firm.

CUCUMBER-PINEAPPLE-GELATIN SALAD

Exchanges per serving: ½ cup = ½ Fruit
Calories per serving: 23   Yield: 3½ cups

1 envelope diet lemon or
   orange gelatin
½ cup hot water
1 cup artificially sweetened
   pineapple tidbits with
   juice

¼ cup lemon or orange
   juice
⅛ teaspoon salt
1½ cups cucumber,
   shredded and drained

Dissolve gelatin in hot water. Drain pineapple, reserving ¼ cup
juice. Add pineapple liquid, lemon or orange juice, and salt to
gelatin. Chill until thickened and consistency of syrup. Fold in
pineapple and cucumber. Pour into 1 quart mold and chill.

LAURA'S JELLIED VEGETABLE SALAD

Exchanges per serving: 1 serving = ½ Vegetable
Calories per serving: 18   Yield: 8 servings

2 envelopes unflavored
gelatin
½ cup cold water
3 cups boiling water
½ cup fresh lemon juice
Nonnutritive sweetener
equivalent to ⅔ cup
sugar

1 tablespoon tarragon
vinegar
1 teaspoon salt
½ cucumber, diced fine
8 or 9 radishes, sliced
8 or 9 scallions, sliced

Soften gelatin in cold water, add boiling water, stir to dissolve.
Blend in lemon juice, sweetener, vinegar, salt, and coloring;
chill until mixture begins to thicken. Fold in vegetables and
place in a lightly oiled 1½ quart mold. Chill until set.

SEAFOOD SALAD

Exchanges per serving: ½ cup = 1½ Fat, 3 Very Lean Meat
Calories per serving: 250   Yield: 4 servings

½ pound deveined shrimp,
shelled, cooked, chilled,
and cut in 2″ pieces
1 tablespoon green onion,
minced
3 tablespoons diet salad
dressing
3 tablespoons diet French
dressing

½ cup chopped almonds
1 cup low-fat cottage
cheese
2 cups lettuce, torn up
1 tomato, cut in wedges
1 teaspoon parsley sprigs,
chopped fine

Mix first six ingredients. Divide evenly on lettuce; garnish with
tomato and parsley.

MEAT or SEAFOOD SALAD
(Suitable for salads or sandwich fillings)

Exchanges per serving: 3 tablespoons = 1 Fat,
1 Very Lean Meat

Calories per serving: 75   Yield: 3 cups

2 cups minced meat,
shellfish, or flaked fish

1 tablespoon green onion,
minced

¼ cup celery, minced

1 teaspoon pimento,
minced

1 teaspoon fresh parsley,
minced, or parsley flakes

1 egg, hard cooked,
chopped fine

1 teaspoon capers, minced

½ cup diet mayonnaise or
diet salad dressing

Salt and pepper to taste

Garlic salt to taste

Combine first seven ingredients. Mix with mayonnaise or salad
dressing; season to taste. Chill.

SUGGESTIONS: Serve as sandwich filling with plain bread or
toasted bun.

Serve as main-plate salad:

1. On bed of chopped lettuce, garnished with curled strips
   of carrot.
2. Stuffed in tomato or avocado.

EASY SALAD DRESSING

Exchanges per serving: 1 tablespoon = None
Calories per serving: 6   Yield: 1¼ cups

1 egg, well beaten

½ teaspoon salt

Dash of pepper

½ teaspoon dry mustard

½ cup vinegar

¼ cup skim milk

Nonnutritive sweetener
equivalent to ½ cup
sugar

Mix all ingredients except sweetener; cook until mixture comes to a racing boil, over low heat. Add sweetener, cool. Use for salads.

VINEGAR DRESSING

Exchanges per serving: 1 tablespoon = None
Calories per serving: 0   Yield: ⅓ cup

¼ cup vinegar
2 tablespoons water
1 clove garlic, crushed
⅙ teaspoon salt
⅛ teaspoon paprika

Nonnutritive sweetener
  equivalent to 3½
  teaspoons sugar
½ teaspoon dill or tarragon
  or a combination of
  rosemary and thyme

Combine all ingredients. Store in jar in refrigerator. Shake well before using.

NONFAT MILK DRESSING

Exchanges per serving: 1 tablespoon = None
Calories per serving: 4   Yield: 3 cups

1 cup white vinegar
Nonnutritive sweetener
  equivalent to ¾ cup
  sugar

2 cups nonfat milk

Beat all ingredients thoroughly with rotary beater. Store in refrigerator. May be used for lettuce, coleslaw, and so on.

SALLY'S SALAD DRESSING

Exchanges per serving: 1 tablespoon = None
Calories per serving: 2   Yield: 3 ounces or 5 tablespoons

2 teaspoons minced onion
4 tablespoons malt or cider
  vinegar

Nonnutritive sweetener
  equivalent to ½ cup
  sugar
2 teaspoons seasoned salt
½ teaspoon lemon pepper

Mix all ingredients well. Serve on fruit or vegetable salads or for coleslaw mix.

FRUIT SALAD DRESSING

Exchanges per serving: 1 tablespoon = None
Calories per serving: 3   Yield: ¾ cup

Nonnutritive sweetener
  equivalent to 3 cups
  sugar
½ cup unsweetened lemon
  juice
½ cup water

½ tablespoon arrowroot
½ teaspoon celery seed
½ teaspoon chervil
1 teaspoon celery salt
½ teaspoon dry mustard
½ teaspoon paprika

Combine sweetener, lemon juice, water, and arrowroot in a small pan; stir to blend. Add remaining ingredients and bring to a boil, cooking until thick and clear (about 3–4 minutes), stirring constantly. Cool; store in refrigerator.

LOW-CALORIE DRESSING

Exchanges per serving: 2 tablespoons = None
Calories per serving: 14   Yield: 1½ cups

1¼ cups condensed tomato
  soup
¼ teaspoon onion salt
⅛ teaspoon black pepper

¼ teaspoon garlic powder
3 tablespoons wine vinegar
1 tablespoon corn relish

Mix all ingredients together in large jar. Cover and refrigerate. Shake before using.

DRESSING À LA BLANCHE

Exchanges per serving: 1 tablespoon = None
Calories per serving: 4   Yield: 3 cups

1 cup white vinegar
2 cups skim milk

Nonnutritive sweetener
   equivalent to ¾ cup
   sugar

Place all ingredients in covered glass jar, shake until well mixed. Store in refrigerator. Use for lettuce, coleslaw, and so on.

MARGE'S SALAD DRESSING

Exchanges per serving: 1 tablespoon = None
Calories per serving: 7   Yield: 1½ cups

1 egg, well beaten
Nonnutritive sweetener
   equivalent to ⅔ cup
   sugar
⅔ cup nonfat milk

½ cup malt vinegar
1 teaspoon mustard
½ teaspoon salt
⅛ teaspoon pepper
½ teaspoon diet margarine

Combine all ingredients in top of double boiler and cook over hot water. Stir until thick and smooth. Chill. Use for vegetable salads.

GOURMET SOUR CREAM DRESSING

Exchanges per serving: 1 tablespoon = ⅓ Fat
Calories per serving: 25   Yield: 1¼ cups

2 tablespoons green onion, minced
3 tablespoons wine vinegar
Nonnutritive sweetener equivalent to 2 tablespoons sugar
1 teaspoon prepared mustard
⅛ teaspoon pepper
Dash of Tabasco sauce
1 cup low-calorie sour cream (calories = 17 per tablespoon with sour half-and-half)

Combine all ingredients. Chill at least 30 minutes to blend flavors.

GINNY'S SALAD DRESSING

Exchanges per serving: 1 tablespoon = None
Calories per serving: 0   Yield: 5 tablespoons

2 teaspoons onion juice
4 tablespoons cider vinegar
Nonnutritive sweetener equivalent to ½ cup sugar
⅛ teaspoon dry mustard
⅛ teaspoon pepper
⅛ teaspoon salt

Mix all ingredients well. Serve on fruit or vegetable salads or for coleslaw mix.

FRUIT DRESSING

Exchanges per serving: 1 tablespoon = ½ Fat
Calories per serving: 21   Yield: 3 cups

¼ teaspoon dry mustard
¼ teaspoon salt
1 teaspoon onion juice
1 cup cider vinegar
4 teaspoons paprika
4 tablespoons celery seed
1½ cups water
½ cup oil
Nonnutritive sweetener equivalent to 3 cups sugar

Combine first five ingredients. Bring to boil; simmer over low heat about 5 minutes; remove from heat. Add remaining ingredients. Chill. Serve on fruit salads.

LOUISE'S SALAD DRESSING

Exchanges per serving: 1 tablespoon = ½ Fat
Calories per serving: 17   Yield: 1 cup

3 egg yolks, beaten well
2 tablespoons nonfat milk
Nonnutritive sweetener
  equivalent to ½ cup
  sugar
½ cup fresh lemon juice
2 teaspoons diet
  margarine, melted
⅛ teaspoon salt

Mix all ingredients in saucepan; cook over medium heat, stirring constantly, until mixture comes to a boil and is slightly thick. Chill.

BLUE CHEESE TOPPING

Exchanges per serving: 1 tablespoon = None
Calories per serving: 9   Yield: 2¼ cups

2 cups plain low-fat yogurt
3 tablespoons low-calorie
  blue cheese dressing
½ teaspoon salt

Combine ingredients; chill. Serve on lettuce leaves or baked potato.

SALAD DRESSING

Exchanges per serving: 1 tablespoon = None
Calories per serving: 8   Yield: 2 cups

2 eggs, well beaten   1 cup malt or cider vinegar
1 teaspoon salt   1 cup nonfat milk
⅛ teaspoon lemon pepper   Nonnutritive sweetener
1 teaspoon dry mustard   equivalent to 1 cup sugar

Mix first six ingredients. Cook until mixture comes to a racing
boil, over low heat. Add sweetener; cool.

CHUTNEY (OR CURRY) MAYONNAISE

Exchanges per serving: 1½ teaspoons = 1 Fat
Calories per serving: 48   Yield: 1 cup

1 cup safflower   1 teaspoon chutney or
   mayonnaise   curry powder
1 teaspoon any minced
   fruit

Blend all ingredients together for spicy sauce for seafoods and
chicken salad.

FRENCH-STYLE VINEGAR DRESSING

Exchanges per serving: 1 tablespoon = 1½ Fat
Calories per serving: 65   Yield: ¾ cup

2 tablespoons vinegar   ½ onion, grated fine
½ teaspoon salt   6 tablespoons oil
1 teaspoon paprika   Nonnutritive sweetener
4 tablespoons lemon juice   equivalent to 1 cup sugar

Bring vinegar, salt, paprika, lemon juice, and onion to a boil.
Cool. Add oil and sweetener; cook again until thick as desired.

THOUSAND ISLAND DRESSING

Exchanges per serving: 1 tablespoon = None
Calories per serving: 9   Yield: 1⅓ cups

1 cup unflavored low-fat
  yogurt
¼ cup catsup (see Index
  for recipe)
2 tablespoons celery, diced
  fine
1 tablespoon green pepper,
  diced fine

1 tablespoon onion,
  chopped fine
Nonnutritive sweetener
  equivalent to ½ cup
  sugar
¼ teaspoon seasoned salt
¼ teaspoon pepper

Mix all ingredients; blend well. Chill overnight in refrigerator.

LUAU MAYONNAISE

Exchanges per serving: 1 tablespoon = 2 Fat
Calories per serving: 80   Yield: 1¼ cups

1 cup safflower
  mayonnaise
2 tablespoons artificially
  sweetened pineapple
  juice

1 tablespoon maraschino
  cherry syrup

Thin mayonnaise with juice and syrup; blend to smooth pink color.

DOTTIE'S FRENCH DRESSING

Exchanges per serving: 1 tablespoon = 2 Fat
Calories per serving: 90   Yield: ¾ cup

½ cup olive oil
¼ cup malt vinegar
¼ teaspoon dry mustard

1 teaspoon salt
Dash of paprika
Dash of lemon pepper

Place all ingredients in glass jar. Blend or shake until well mixed. Chill.

CHEESE AND EGG DISHES

NOTES

Cheeses, for the most part, are high in fat content since they are made from whole milk, often with cream added. See Meat Exchange List for categorized cheese choices. *Example:* Cheddar is a High-Fat Meat, whereas part-skim milk mozzarella is a Medium-Fat Meat.

Wherever possible, bread and cereal products should be whole grain. Fiber is an important component in the diet. Recent research indicates that including fiber in the diet assists in the control of blood sugar.

The following cheeses are available in some areas; check your market:

Neufchâtel Cream Cheese: 3 tablespoons = 23 calories

*Golden Image Mild Imitation Cheddar Cheese: 1 ounce = 57 calories

*Golden Image Imitation Colby Cheese: 1 ounce = 55 calories

*Philadelphia Brand Imitation Cream Cheese: 1 ounce = 52 calories

Tasty Brand Imitation Pasteurized Processed Cheese Spread: 1 ounce = 75 calories

*Golden Image Imitation Pasteurized Processed Cheese Spread: 1 ounce = 48 calories

*Golden Image Imitation Pasteurized Processed Food Singles: 1¾-ounce slice = 38 calories

You may also find:

Kraft Low Calorie Imitation Grape Jelly: 1 tablespoon = 12 calories

* Indicates limited distribution.

Kraft Low Calorie Imitation Strawberry Preserves: 1 tablespoon = 14 calories

Fried eggs and omelets can be cooked beautifully in a
Teflon-coated pan without the addition of fat.

When using basic ingredients such as arrowroot, eggs, flour,
margarine, and tapioca, refer to Weights, Measures, and the
Metric System, Notes on Special Ingredients Used in Recipes,
and Additional Suggestions (see Contents).

FLUFF OMELET

Exchanges per serving: 1 serving = 1 Medium-Fat Meat
Calories per serving: 75   Yield: 1 serving

| 1 egg | Dash of salt |
| 1 tablespoon water | |

Using a wire whisk, beat all ingredients together. Place in
Teflon pan and cook until done.

VARIATIONS: Diet Jelly: No additional calories.
Cheese: ½ ounce grated cheese, add 35 calories to above. Ham
and Green Pepper: 1 tablespoon ham and 1½ tablespoons
chopped green pepper, add 35 calories to above.

EGGS CURRY

Exchanges per serving: 1 serving = 1 Starch, 1½ Medium-Fat
                               Meat, ½ Fat, ½ Nonfat Milk,
                               ¼ Vegetable

Calories per serving: 275   Yield: 4 servings

6 eggs, hard-boiled	1½ tablespoons arrowroot
¼ cup almonds, slivered	1 teaspoon salt
2 tablespoons diet margarine	1½ teaspoons curry powder
1 onion, chopped fine	2 cups nonfat milk
½ cup celery, chopped fine	4 slices toast

Thinly slice shelled eggs. Brown almonds in margarine until golden brown. Remove; drain on absorbent paper. In same pan sauté onion and celery until golden; stir in arrowroot, salt, and curry powder; stir in milk slowly. Cook, stirring constantly, until thick and smooth. Stir in sliced egg; heat to boil. Place a slice of toast in the bottom of each of four individual heated casseroles. Divide eggs evenly over the toast; sprinkle with almonds.

SCRAMBLED EGGS

Exchanges per serving: 1 serving = 1 Medium-Fat Meat
Calories per serving: 78   Yield: 1 serving

1 egg	Salt
1 tablespoon nonfat milk	Pepper

To eliminate the use of fat, scramble eggs in double boiler (or use Teflon-coated pan). Mix egg and milk with wire whip or fork; add salt and pepper, and for variety, a dash of curry powder or chopped chives, green onion, or parsley. For a spicy variation, add 2 tablespoons salsa to raw egg mixture, then cook.

OMELET WITH COTTAGE CHEESE

Exchanges per serving: 1 serving = 1 Fat, 2 Medium-Fat Meat,
                                            1 Very Lean Meat
Calories per serving: 240   Yield: 2 servings

2 tablespoons diet margarine	½ cup low-fat cottage cheese, sieved
4 eggs, separated	Dash of pepper
Dash of salt	1 tablespoon chervil

Preheat over to 350°F. Melt margarine in skillet. Beat egg whites with salt until stiff but not dry. Beat yolks separately until lemon-colored and thick; add cheese and pepper and beat until smooth. Fold in egg whites and chervil. Place mixture in skillet; cook over medium heat until lightly browned on bottom and fluffy (about 3–4 minutes). Place in oven 15 minutes; make a crease down center with knife and fold over. Serve at once.

EGGS ON TOAST, OVEN STYLE

Exchanges per serving: 1 serving = 1 Starch, ⅓ Fat,
                                            1 Medium-Fat Meat
Calories per serving: 157   Yield: 6 servings

6 slices bread	1 tablespoon chervil
6 teaspoons diet margarine	⅛ teaspoon salt
6 eggs, separated	⅛ teaspoon pepper

Preheat oven to 350°F. Butter each slice of bread with margarine; place buttered-side-up on cookie sheet. Beat egg whites until stiff; distribute evenly on bread slices. Make a hollow in center of each; fill with yolk. Sprinkle eggs with chervil, salt, and pepper. Bake until yolk is nearly set and white is lightly browned (about 15 minutes). Serve at once.

EGGS WITH CHEESE SAUCE

Exchanges per serving: 1 egg with ¼ cup sauce and 1 slice of
      toast = 1 Starch, 1 Medium-Fat Meat, ¾ High-Fat Meat
Calories per serving: 230   Yield: 6 servings, 4 cups sauce*

1¼ tablespoons arrowroot	1 tablespoon diet
½ teaspoon salt	margarine
Dash of cayenne	1½ cups (5 ounces)
1 tablespoon prepared	cheddar cheese, grated
mustard	6 eggs
1 tablespoon chervil	6 slices bread
½ cup nonfat milk	

Preheat oven to 350°F. Butter individual custard cups. Mix first
five ingredients together; stir in milk slowly. Continue stirring
over medium heat until thick and smooth. Remove from heat;
stir in margarine and cheese. Stir until cheese has melted and
sauce is smooth. Break one egg into each cup; cover with ¼ cup
cheese sauce. Bake until firm (15–20 minutes). Toast bread; cut
in half; serve egg with toast.

CHEESE TOAST AND EGGS

Exchanges per serving: 1 serving = 1 Starch,
                        2 Medium-Fat Meat
Calories per serving: 230   Yield: 4 servings

4 slices bread	4 eggs, poached
4 ounces mozzarella	
cheese	

Preheat over to 350°F. Toast bread; top each slice with 1 oz.
cheese. Put on cookie sheet; place in oven until cheese just melts
(2–3 minutes). Add poached egg on top. Serve at once.

* Refrigerate balance of sauce for use another time.

SALLY'S CHEESE FONDUE
(Not for diabetics without consent of doctor)

Exchanges per serving: 1 slice = 1 Starch, ⅔ High-Fat Meat
Calories per serving: 168   Yield: 12 servings

1 clove garlic, peeled
2 cups dry white wine
2 cups cheese, shredded
  fine*
¼ teaspoon arrowroot
2 tablespoons
  Kirschwasser

Dash of pepper
Dash of salt
Dash of nutmeg
12 slices firm bread, cut
  into cubes, leaving one
  side of crust on each cube

Rub an earthenware casserole with garlic, then add wine. Heat slowly over chafing dish burner. Mix cheese lightly with arrowroot; when bubbles in wine rise to surface, add cheese mix a handful at a time. Stir each handful until it melts; continue until all cheese is melted. Add Kirschwasser and seasonings; stir well. Turn heat low but keep fondue slowly bubbling. Have each person take a cube of bread on the end of a fork and twirl it in the bubbling fondue. If fondue is too thick, add a little *hot* wine.

---

* This could be Swiss cheese made with skim milk.

HAM AND CHEESE ON BUNS

Exchanges per serving: ½ bun = 1 Starch, 2 Lean Meat
Calories per serving: 193   Yield: 6 servings

3 hamburger buns, sliced
across

6 1-ounce slices baked ham

¼ cup dietetic cranberry
sauce

6 1-ounce slices skim-milk
mozzarella cheese or 6
ounces cheese, grated,
divided into 6 servings

Toast bun halves slightly; top each with slice of ham. Spread
each with cranberry sauce; place thin slice of cheese (or 1 ounce
grated) over this; put under broiler until cheese melts and is
lightly browned.

BLINTZES WITH CHEESE FILLING

Exchanges per serving: 1 blintz = ½ Starch, ¾ Very Lean Meat,
                                  ¼ Medium-Fat Meat
Calories per serving: 100   Yield: 1 dozen

1 cup flour
½ teaspoon salt
½ teaspoon baking powder
1 cup nonfat milk
3 eggs
2 tablespoons diet
margarine, melted

2 cups low-fat cottage
cheese, sieved
Nonnutritive sweetener
equivalent to 2
tablespoons sugar
½ teaspoon cinnamon
¼ teaspoon allspice or
nutmeg

Sift flour, salt, and baking powder together. Beat milk, 2 eggs,
and margarine. Slowly add to flour mixture; stir to form thin
batter. Grease frying pan lightly, then pour ⅛ cup (2 tablespoons) batter into skillet; tilt skillet to cover bottom completely.
Cook until top of pancake is firm; turn onto paper towel, with
uncooked side down on waxed paper. Make rest of pancakes,
greasing skillet as necessary. Mix cottage cheese, sweetener, cinnamon, allspice or nutmeg, and remaining egg. Top each pan-

cake with a tablespoon of filling. Fold over sides, then the ends, to make small drugstore-type package; set to one side. Refrigerate until ready to serve. A few minutes before serving, melt margarine in skillet and lightly brown each blintz, starting with flap side down. Turn and brown on other side. Serve warm.

FISH, MEAT, AND POULTRY

CHOP SUEY WITH TUNA

Exchanges per serving: 1 cup = 1 Starch, 1 Lean Meat
Calories per serving: 130   Yield: 4 servings

2 stalks celery, cut small
½ onion, chopped fine
2 cups + 2 tablespoons
   water
¾ cup rice
Nonnutritive sweetener
   equivalent to ½ teaspoon
   sugar

Dash of pepper
2 tablespoons soy sauce
¾ cup water-packed tuna,
   drained (or any cooked
   poultry could be
   substituted for a
   different dish)

Cook celery and onion in 2 tablespoons water over low heat, covered. When tender, remove from heat; add rice, 2 cups water, and seasonings; bring to boil. Turn heat low and cook, covered, until rice is tender and liquid absorbed (about 30 minutes). Add tuna. Mix and remove from heat; set aside, covered, for a few minutes before serving.

NOTE: If desired, you can add ⅔ cup of canned, fresh, or frozen chop suey vegetables for more nutrition. This would add 35 calories per serving.

CHEESE AND CRAB ORIENTAL STYLE

Exchanges per serving: 1 serving = ¼ Starch, 2 Very Lean
Meat, ½ High-Fat Meat,
2 Vegetable, 1 Fat

Calories per serving: 225   Yield: 5 servings

½ cup mushrooms, sliced
½ carrot, sliced thin
¼ cup green pepper, diced
1 cup celery, sliced
1 cup onion, chopped fine
2 tablespoons oil
Nonnutritive sweetener
  equivalent to
  1 tablespoon sugar

1 teaspoon salt
1 bay leaf
4 cups tomatoes, fresh or
  canned
¾ cup rice, precooked
1½ cups crab meat, frozen,
  thawed, and drained
½ cup sharp cheese, grated

Preheat oven to 350°F. Sauté first five ingredients in oil in
Dutch oven or other ovenproof container until onion is golden
brown. Add sweetener, salt, bay leaf, and tomatoes; boil for 5
minutes, gently. Stir in rice and crab meat. Sprinkle entire mixture with grated cheese. Bake 20–25 minutes.

FISH AND MUSHROOMS

Exchanges per serving: 1 serving = ¾ Fat, 4 Very Lean Meat,
1 Vegetable

Calories per serving: 200   Yield: 4 servings

1 onion, sliced thin	Dash of salt
1 tablespoon oil	Dash of pepper
1½ cups mushrooms, sliced thin	1 stalk celery, sliced thin
1 pound fish fillets (cod, halibut, sole) cut in 1″ slices	1 tablespoon soy sauce
	1 tablespoon dry sherry

Preheat skillet and sauté onion in oil. Add mushrooms and sauté about 2 minutes, stirring constantly, until mushrooms wilt. Spread half of fillet slices on mushrooms; sprinkle with salt and pepper, add remaining fillets; sprinkle these with salt and pepper. Add celery, soy sauce, and sherry; cook gently, covered, for 10 minutes.

HARRIET'S FISH DISH

Exchanges per serving: 1 serving = ¼ Fat, 4 Very Lean Meat,
2 Vegetable

Calories per serving: 220   Yield: 4 servings

2 onions, sliced thin	2 cups canned tomatoes
1 clove garlic, crushed	1 tablespoon tomato paste
1 tablespoon diet margarine	2 chicken bouillon cubes
½ cup parsley, snipped	4 4-ounce fish fillets or steaks, about ¾″ thick
½ teaspoon salt	3 slices tomato, cut thin
⅛ teaspoon pepper	3 slices lemon, cut thin

Preheat over to 300°F. Sauté onions and garlic in margarine until golden; add parsley, salt, pepper, tomatoes with juice, tomato paste, and bouillon cubes. Simmer gently, uncovered, about 20 minutes. Place fish steaks in medium baking dish. Cover with sauce; top with tomato slices and lemons. Bake until tender.

BAKED FISH STEAKS

Exchanges per serving: 3 ounces = ¾ Fat, 3 Very Lean Meat,
¼ Starch, ¼ Vegetable

Calories per serving: 180   Yield: 4 servings

4 3-ounce fish steaks   ½ carrot, sliced thin
  (halibut, swordfish, or   Dash of salt
  similar)   Dash of pepper
3 teaspoons oil   ½ teaspoon parsley,
1 onion, sliced thin   snipped
1 potato, sliced thin

Preheat oven to 450°F. Remove skin from fish steaks; cut meat
away from bone. Cut four 10″ × 12″ pieces of heavy duty foil, use
oil to grease center of each piece of foil; place a steak on each
piece of foil. Top each steak with slices of onion, potato, carrot,
and salt and pepper. Using drugstore folds, wrap each piece separately. Put on cookie sheet and bake until fish flakes and is tender, approximately 20 minutes. Garnish with parsley.

HILO FILLET OF SOLE

Exchanges per serving: 3 ounces = 4 Fat, 3 Very Lean Meat
Calories per serving: 355   Yield: 8 servings

1½ pounds fish fillets (cod, halibut, sole)
¼ teaspoon salt
2 teaspoons instant minced onion
1½ teaspoons water
¾ cup safflower mayonnaise
1 teaspoon lemon juice
¼ teaspoon seasoned salt
1 teaspoon parsley, finely chopped
⅓ cup chopped macadamia nuts or slivered almonds

Wipe fillets with damp cloth; sprinkle with salt. Roll and secure each with toothpick. Place rolls in steamer or on wire rack above boiling water; cover and steam 15 minutes. Mix onion, water, mayonnaise, lemon juice, seasoned salt, and parsley. Remove fillets carefully from steamer; spread quickly with mayonnaise mixture. Top with nuts and serve at once.

SHRIMP AND RICE

Exchanges per serving: ½ cup rice and ¾ cup sauce = 1 Starch,
                        3½ Very Lean Meat, 1 Vegetable
Calories per serving: 280   Yield: 4 servings

2 cups tomatoes
2 tablespoons parsley flakes
2 cups celery, sliced thin
¼ teaspoon basil
1½ teaspoons salt
⅛ teaspoon pepper
½ teaspoon oregano
3-ounce can tomato paste
2 7-ounce packages frozen, deveined, shelled shrimp
½ cup long-grain rice

Mix everything except shrimp and rice in large skillet, stirring occasionally. Boil gently, uncovered, until celery is nearly tender (about 30 minutes). Stir in shrimp; boil until shrimp are cooked but still tender (about 5–10 minutes). Cook rice as directed, omitting margarine or butter. Serve shrimp over rice.

CRAB, SHRIMP, RICE SUPREME
(Moderate cholesterol)

Exchanges per serving: ¾ cup = ½ Starch, 1½ Fat,
1½ Very Lean Meat

Calories per serving: 228   Yield: 10 servings

2 cups cooked rice
1 cup diet mayonnaise
½ cup green onion,
chopped
¼ cup green pepper,
chopped
1 cup tomato juice

¼ cup toasted almonds,
slivered
8 ounces fresh, frozen, or
canned crab meat
8 ounces fresh, frozen, or
canned shrimp
¼ cup prepared bread
crumbs

Preheat oven to 350°F. Mix all ingredients except bread crumbs
together; place in casserole and top with bread crumbs. Bake 1
hour. Use fresh seafood if available. This is an excellent party
casserole as it can be made a day ahead and refrigerated.

TUNA (OR SALMON) PIE WITH CRUST

Exchanges per serving: 1 serving = 1 Bread, ⅓ Fat, 2 Medium-
Fat Meat, 1 High-Fat Meat

Calories per serving: 345   Yield: 6 servings

1 cup long-grain white rice, uncooked	¼ teaspoon salt
2 tablespoons diet margarine	⅛ teaspoon pepper
3 eggs	⅛ teaspoon nutmeg
1¼ cups water-packed tuna (or pink salmon), drained and flaked	¾ cup American cheese, grated
	¾ cup nonfat milk, scalded
	½ teaspoon parsley

Preheat oven to 400°F. Cook rice as directed; mix with margarine and one egg. Line a 9″ pie pan with rice mix; mound rice
mixture up to about 1″ above rim of plate. Spread tuna (or
salmon) in shell; sprinkle with salt, pepper, nutmeg, and cheese.
Beat remaining eggs in small bowl; stir in scalded milk. Return
to pan and heat until smooth; pour mixture over cheese. Bake
until cheese is dark golden brown (about 30 minutes). Sprinkle
parsley over top.

SALMON (OR TUNA) CASSEROLE

Exchanges per serving: ½ cup = ¼ Starch, ½ Fat, 1½ Lean Meat
Calories per serving: 140   Yield: 24 ½-cup servings

1 cup dry noodles, uncooked	½ cup flour
2 cups mushrooms, sliced thin	2 teaspoons paprika
4 tablespoons onion, chopped fine	2 cups nonfat milk
4 tablespoons diet margarine	2 cups half-and-half
1 teaspoon salt	4 cups pink salmon (or tuna, water-packed and well drained)
¼ teaspoon pepper	1 cup Parmesan cheese, grated

Preheat oven to 375°F. Cook noodles according to directions on the package. Sauté mushrooms and onion in margarine until tender, stir in salt, pepper, flour, and paprika. Stir in milk slowly, cooking and stirring constantly until thick and smooth. Remove from heat; stir in half-and-half. Remove skin and bones from drained salmon (or tuna), then flake. Mix fish with noodles, mushroom mixture, and all but a little of the grated cheese. Pour into casserole; sprinkle remaining cheese on top. Bake 20–25 minutes.

SWEET-SOUR TONGUE

Exchanges per serving: 1 ounce = 1 Very Lean Meat, ½ Fat
Calories per serving: 90   Yield: 3 servings

2 tablespoons diet
    margarine
1 tablespoon arrowroot
½ teaspoon salt
Nonnutritive sweetener
    equivalent to 2
    tablespoons sugar

2 tablespoons malt vinegar
¼ teaspoon pepper
1 cup stock
3 ounces cooked smoked
    tongue, sliced

Blend first six ingredients with stock; cook until thickened. Add tongue and heat.

STUFFED BUNS

Exchanges per serving: 1 bun = 2 Starch, 1 Fat, ¾ Medium-Fat
Meat, ¼ High-Fat Meat

Calories per serving: 285   Yield: 8 servings

6-ounce can diet water-
packed tuna (or chicken
or turkey)
2 tablespoons green onion,
minced
2 tablespoons celery,
minced

1 tablespoon ripe olives,
chopped
Minced dill pickle to taste
½ cup diet mayonnaise
¼ cup cheddar cheese,
grated
8 frankfurter buns

Mix first seven ingredients; fill buns with mixture. Wrap in foil.
Place in 350°F oven about 10–15 minutes until hot and cheese
has melted.

ONION, LIVER, AND CHEESE
(High cholesterol)

Exchanges per serving: 2 ounces liver = ⅓ Fat, 2 Lean Meat
1 tablespoon cheddar cheese =
½ High-Fat Meat

Calories per serving: 175   Yield: 6 servings

1 pound beef liver,
quartered
1 tablespoon flour
Dash of salt
Dash of pepper
Dash of garlic salt

2 tablespoons diet
margarine
½ cup cheddar cheese,
grated
1 onion, sliced very thin

Remove skin and veins from beef liver; cut into ½″ serving
pieces. Sprinkle lightly with flour; shake off excess and sprinkle
salt, pepper, and garlic salt on each side. Sauté liver in margarine a few minutes over medium heat. Turn off heat. Pour off
most of margarine; return pan to burner; sprinkle pieces with
cheese, then thin rounds of onion. Cover; heat until cheese is
melted. Serve.

LIVER À LA BOURGEOISE
(High cholesterol)

Exchanges per serving: 3½–4 ounces = ¼ Fat, 3–4 Lean Meat,
½ Vegetable

Calories per serving: 215   Yield: 8 servings

1 carrot, shredded	1 tablespoon arrowroot
1 onion, minced	2½ pounds beef liver*
1 turnip, diced	2 cups water
1 bay leaf	Dash of seasoned salt
2 tablespoons diet margarine	Dash of lemon pepper

Brown carrot, onion, and turnip with the bay leaf in margarine.
Add arrowroot and blend. Add liver and water. Season and
simmer 1½ to 1¾ hours.

FRANKFURTER CASSEROLE

Exchanges per serving: 1 serving = 1 Starch, 1 Fat, ¼ High-Fat
Meat, ⅓ Vegetable

Calories per serving: 160   Yield: 8 servings

1¼ cups condensed bean and bacon soup	1 green pepper, chopped fine
1¼ cups water	½ cup celery, chopped fine
2 all-beef frankfurters (or chicken or turkey franks), cut into ½" pieces	2 tablespoons prepared mustard
1 onion, chopped fine	1 can ready-mix biscuit mixture, prepared as package directs

Preheat oven to 375°F. Mix all ingredients except biscuits. Boil
gently 5 minutes. Put 3 pieces of frankfurter into each of 8 individual baking dishes; add about ¾ cup mixture; top each with
biscuit. Bake until biscuits are dark golden brown (about 20
minutes). Serve at once.

* Note: 5 oz. with shrinkage = 3½–4 oz. servings.

CALIFORNIA POT ROAST

Exchanges per serving: 2 ounces meat = 2 Lean Meat
Calories per serving: 125   Yield: 20 servings

4 pounds beef rump roast	1 tablespoon
2 tablespoons flour	Worcestershire sauce
1 teaspoon salt	1 cup water
Dash of pepper	Nonnutritive sweetener
1 tablespoon oil	equivalent to ½ cup
1 onion, chopped fine	sugar
2 carrots, sliced	

Dredge meat well in flour, salt, and pepper. Brown in oil in skillet; add remaining ingredients. Cover; simmer about 4 hours over low heat.

ROAST BEEF WITH FRUIT SAUCE

Exchanges per serving: 1 ounce = 1 Lean Meat
                       ¼ cup sauce = 1 Fruit
Calories per serving: 43 (sauce), 55 (meat)   Yield: 3 cups sauce

3- to 4-pound rump round/sirloin-cut roast (lean meat group)	Salt and pepper to taste

Trim fat from beef before roasting. Salt and pepper. Place roast on rack; bake at 325°F for 1½ hours. Trim remaining fat after roasting.

SAUCE

4 cups artificially sweetened plums (reserve syrup)	⅓ cup unsweetened frozen orange juice concentrate
¼ teaspoon salt	2 tablespoons
⅛ teaspoon pepper	Worcestershire sauce
1 tablespoon arrowroot	⅛ teaspoon Tabasco sauce

Drain and pit plums. Save ¾ cup syrup. Puree plums until smooth; add syrup and remaining ingredients. Blend until smooth. In medium saucepan, heat to boiling. Serve over roast beef.

HAMBURGER CORNMEAL SHEPHERD'S PIE

Exchanges per serving: 1 serving = 1 Starch, 2 Fat, 2 Medium-
Fat Meat, ⅓ Vegetable

Calories per serving: 330   Yield: 8 servings

½ cup green pepper, chopped fine

¼ cup onion, minced fine

16 ounces (1 lb.) lean ground round (15 percent fat)

5 tablespoons oil

1 cup tomato sauce

2 tablespoons low-calorie catsup (see Index)

2 teaspoons salt

Dash of lemon pepper

1 teaspoon chili powder

½ cup flour, sifted

¾ cup yellow cornmeal

Nonnutritive sweetener equivalent to 1 tablespoon sugar

2 teaspoons baking powder

½ teaspoon thyme

1 egg

½ cup nonfat milk

Preheat oven to 400°F. Sauté green pepper, onion, and beef in 2 tablespoons oil in skillet, until beef is well browned. Stir in tomato sauce, catsup, 1 teaspoon salt, lemon pepper, and chili powder. Put into 1½ quart casserole. Stir flour, cornmeal, sweetener, baking powder, remaining salt, and thyme together in a bowl; add egg, milk, and remaining oil. Stir until smooth. Top the first mixture with the second; bake uncovered, until cornbread is slightly brown and firm to touch (about 30 minutes). Loosen cornbread with a knife around edges; turn onto serving plate with top side down.

MEAT CASSEROLE

Exchanges per serving: 4-ounce serving = ½ Starch, 3 Lean
Meat, 2 Vegetable

Calories per serving: 255   Yield: 4 servings
(will vary with meat used)

¾ cup noodles, uncooked   2 cups lean beef, cut in 1″
2½ cups tomato juice   cubes, cooked
2 cups celery, chopped fine   ⅛ teaspoon pepper
½ cup green pepper,   1½ teaspoons salt
chopped fine   ½ teaspoon diet margarine

Heat oven to 350°F. Combine all ingredients; turn into well-greased casserole; bake 45 minutes.

SPAGHETTI AND SAUCE

Exchanges per serving: 1 serving = 1 Starch, 3 Lean Meat,
¾ Fat, 1 Vegetable

Calories per serving: 305   Yield: 8 servings sauce;
½ cup cooked spaghetti
per serving

3 cups (1½ pounds) lean   2 tablespoons oil
ground beef (15 percent   ¾ cup tomato paste
fat)   1½ cups tomato juice
1 cup onion, chopped fine   2 teaspoons salt
½ cup celery, chopped fine   Dash of pepper
2 cloves garlic, minced   2 ounces thin spaghetti per
very fine   serving
½ cup fresh mushrooms,
sliced thin

Brown meat well; sauté onion, celery, garlic, and mushrooms in oil until onion is golden brown. Add tomato paste, tomato juice, salt, and pepper; cover; boil gently for 1½ hours. After cooling, refrigerate overnight. About 20 minutes before serving, cook spaghetti according to package instructions; drain thoroughly. Measure sauce and add enough water to make a total of 5 cups of sauce. Return sauce to pan, cover, and boil gently about 10 minutes. Place ½ cup cooked spaghetti on each plate; top with ⅔ cup meat sauce.

CHILI CON CARNE

Exchanges per serving: 1 serving = 1 Starch, 1½ Medium-Fat
Meat, ½ Very Lean Meat
Calories per serving: 208   Yield: 8 servings

- 1 pound coarse ground beef chuck (chili grind)
- 1 cup onion, chopped fine
- 1 clove garlic, crushed fine
- 2 tablespoons chili powder
- 1¼ cups condensed tomato soup
- 2 cups canned kidney beans
- 1 tablespoon malt vinegar
- ¼ teaspoon salt

Brown beef in hot skillet; drain in sieve and pat dry with paper towel; stir in onion, garlic, and chili powder. Cook, stirring often, until onion is tender. Add remaining ingredients; bring to boil. Reduce heat and simmer, uncovered, stirring occasionally, about 15 minutes.

POLLY'S CHILI CON CARNE

Exchanges per serving: 1 serving = 1 Starch, ½ Fat, 4 Very
                                    Lean Meat, 1 Vegetable
Calories per serving: 283   Yield: 5 servings

1 cup onion, chopped fine
½ cup green pepper,
  chopped fine
2 cups celery, chopped fine
1 clove garlic, sliced thin
1 tablespoon oil

2 cups coarse ground
  chuck roast (no added
  fat)
2 cups kidney beans,
  thoroughly drained
2 cups tomatoes
1 tablespoon chili powder
½ teaspoon salt

Sauté onion, pepper, celery, and garlic in oil until onion is
golden brown. Add beef; cook until well browned. Stir in kidney beans, tomatoes, chili powder, and salt; simmer uncovered
about 45–50 minutes. Just before serving, taste to see if more
chili powder is needed.

CORNED BEEF DINNER

Exchanges per serving: 3-ounce slice = ½ Starch, 2 Vegetables,
                                       3 Medium-Fat Meat
Calories per serving: 300   Yield: 16 3-ounce servings

4-pound corned-beef
  round
Water
6 onions
6 carrots

6 parsnips, scraped
3 potatoes (4 ounces each),
  peeled and scraped
6 cups cabbage

Cover meat with cold water in Dutch oven; bring to a boil;
drain. Add water to cover; again bring to boil: reduce heat to
low. Cover. Cook until meat is nearly tender (about 3 hours),
skimming off as much fat as possible from cooking water. (If
you remove meat from broth and refrigerate—or put in freezer,
if time is short—fat will harden and remove easily.) Add vegetables; cook until vegetables are done (about 10–15 minutes

more). Remove vegetables from water; drain, and trim fat from meat.

STUFFED FLANK STEAK

Exchanges per serving: 2 ounces = ¼ Starch, ¼ Fat,
2 Lean Meat

Calories per serving: 145   Yield: 16 servings

2-pound flank steak	¾ cup celery, chopped fine
Dash of salt	1½ teaspoons sage
Dash of lemon pepper	½ teaspoon Mei Yen
1 tablespoon flour	seasoning
4 cups bread cubes	3 tablespoons diet
2 small onions, chopped	margarine
fine	½ cup water

Preheat oven to 350°F. Score steak lightly, crosswise. Sprinkle with salt and lemon pepper; dredge in flour; pound coating well into the steak. Combine next five ingredients; spread over steak. Roll meat and tie, or fasten edge with toothpicks. Brown in margarine, then add water; cover and cook about 1½ hours, until tender. Baste occasionally.

MEAT LOAF

Exchanges per serving: 1 serving = ½ Starch, 2½ Lean Meat
Calories per serving: 190   Yield: 6 servings

1 egg	2 tablespoons green
2 cups lean ground round	pepper, chopped fine
(15 percent fat)	1 teaspoon salt
3 slices bread, cubed fine	½ teaspoon dry mustard
¼ cup catsup (see Index)	1 tablespoon prepared
⅓ cup onion, chopped fine	horseradish, if desired

Preheat oven to 400°F. Mix all ingredients well. Form into a loaf. Place in foil-lined 9″ × 5″ × 3″ pan; bake until done (15–20 minutes).

MEATBALLS WITH CARAWAY SEEDS

Exchanges per serving: 2 meatballs = ¼ Starch, 2 Lean Meat
Calories per serving: 182   Yield: 8 servings

2 cups lean ground round (15 percent fat)	1 tablespoon dried parsley flakes
1 onion, minced fine	8 ounces raw potato coarsely grated
1 egg	2½ cups water
1 teaspoon lemon peel, grated fine	4 beef bouillon cubes
¼ teaspoon pepper	1 teaspoon arrowroot
½ teaspoon salt	½ teaspoon caraway seeds
	1 tablespoon water

Mix first eight ingredients; form into sixteen meatballs. Bring water to boil; dissolve bouillon cubes in water. Add meatballs; cover tightly. Gently boil about 30 minutes. Remove meatballs from broth; stir arrowroot and caraway seeds into 1 tablespoon water; stir into broth until thick and smooth. Pour a little gravy over meatballs; garnish with parsley, if desired. (Store remaining gravy in tightly covered jar in refrigerator for later use.)

MEATBALLS

Exchanges per serving: 2 meatballs = ½ Starch, 1 Lean Meat
Calories per serving: 135   Yield: 12 servings

2 cups lean ground round (15 percent fat)	1½ cups buttermilk
¼ cup prepared bread crumbs	¾ cup instant rice
1 teaspoon salt	1 teaspoon diet margarine
	1 cup water
	½ tablespoon arrowroot

Mix beef, crumbs, salt, ½ cup buttermilk, and rice. Shape into two dozen meatballs (about 1″ round). In large skillet, brown meatballs in margarine on all sides; pour water over; cover tightly. Boil until rice is tender and meat is cooked (about 30 minutes). Remove from skillet. Mix remaining 1 cup buttermilk with arrowroot to form smooth paste; stir into liquid remaining in skillet. Stirring constantly, cook until gravy is thick (do not boil). Return meatballs to pan and gently heat. Serve with gravy.

ROAST LEG OF LAMB

Exchanges per serving: 3 ounces = 3 Lean Meat
Calories per serving: 156   Yield: 10–12 servings

5- to 6-pound leg of lamb	1 teaspoon ginger
1 clove garlic	1 teaspoon seasoned salt
2–3 teaspoons Bouquet Garni	1 teaspoon lemon pepper
	2 tablespoons flour

Preheat oven to 300°F. Wipe meat with damp cloth. Do not remove the fell (the paperlike covering over the meat). Make gashes in roast with sharp knife; cut garlic into slivers and insert a piece in each gash. Rub meat with seasonings; dredge with flour. Place, fat side up, in shallow roaster. Roast uncovered until tender (about 30–35 minutes per pound). Remove garlic and serve.

VEAL À LA KING

Exchanges per serving: 1½ ounces = ½ Starch, 2 Lean Meat,
¼ Skim Milk

Calories per serving: 175   Yield: 16 servings
(3 tablespoons each serving)

½ cup green pepper, chopped fine	4 cups nonfat milk
½ cup mushrooms	Dash of seasoned salt
3 tablespoons diet margarine	Dash of pepper
3 tablespoons arrowroot	4 cups cooked veal, diced
	1 pimento, diced
	8 slices toast

Cook pepper and mushrooms in margarine for 8 minutes; remove vegetables. Add arrowroot to margarine; blend. Add
milk and seasonings; cook until thickened, stirring constantly.
Add green pepper, mushrooms, veal, and pimento; heat. Spoon
3 tablespoons over each ½ slice toast.

SAUERKRAUT AND SPARERIBS

Exchanges per serving: 2 ounces meat and ½ cup sauerkraut =
2 Lean Meat, ½ Vegetable

Calories per serving: 125   Yield: 6 servings

3 cups sauerkraut	4 pounds spareribs*
Nonnutritive sweetener equivalent to ¼ cup brown sugar	Dash of seasoned salt
	Dash of pepper
	½ cup hot water

Preheat oven to 350°F. Place sauerkraut in greased baking dish.
Sprinkle with sweetener. Brown parboiled spareribs under
broiler. Season, place on sauerkraut; add hot water. Cover. Bake
45 minutes to 1 hour.

---

* Approximately 8 ounces including bone, for 2 ounces meat. Parboil ribs to defat as
much as possible.

HAM LOAF

Exchanges per serving: 1 serving = ¼ Starch, 2 Lean Meat
Calories per serving: 140   Yield: 16 servings

1½ pounds lean ham,
  ground well
1 pound lean ground beef
2 eggs, beaten
1¼ cups nonfat milk
4 slices soft bread, broken
  into small pieces
1½ teaspoons salt
Dash of pepper

Nonnutritive sweetener
  equivalent to ¾ cup
  sugar
¼ teaspoon cinnamon
¼ teaspoon cloves
¼ teaspoon nutmeg
½ teaspoon dry mustard
½ teaspoon vegetable oil

Preheat oven to 350°F. Combine all ingredients except oil; mix well. Use oil to grease pan. Place mixture in 2-quart baking dish. Bake 1½ hours.

BAKED HAM OR HAM STEAK WITH PINEAPPLE

Exchanges per serving: 3 ounces = ¼ Fruit, 3 Lean Meat
Calories per serving: 180   Yield: 24 servings

6-pound canned ham
Nonnutritive sweetener
  equivalent to ½ cup
  sugar
1 teaspoon dry mustard

½ cup bread crumbs
¾ cup pineapple juice
5–6 slices unsweetened
  pineapple

Preheat oven to 300°F. Place ham in baking dish. Spread ham with mixture of sweetener, mustard, and bread crumbs. Add pineapple juice. Bake 15 minutes. Add slices of pineapple and cook entire dish an additional 45 minutes.

PORK ROAST WITH SPICE SAUCE

Exchanges per serving: 3 ounces = 3 Lean Meat
Calories per serving: 200   Yield: 12 servings

4-pound fresh pork picnic
    shoulder
Dash of salt
Dash of pepper
2 small onions, minced
1 tablespoon
    Worcestershire sauce

Nonnutritive sweetener
    equivalent to 1½ cups
    sugar
½ teaspoon paprika
½ cup vinegar
½ cup water
2 tablespoons catsup
    (see Index)

Have butcher bone and roll roast. Salt and pepper roast; place
fat side up on rack in open roaster. Roast at 350°F. 40–45 minutes per pound. Combine other ingredients; cook together for 5
minutes. Pour over roast and serve.

PORK PATTIES IN GRAVY

Exchanges per serving: 1 serving = ½ Starch, 1 Fat, 2 Lean
                                    Meat, 1 Vegetable
Calories per serving: 225   Yield: 8 servings

2 cups very lean pork
    shoulder, trimmed of all
    visible fat, then ground
2 eggs
½ cup nonfat milk
4 slices dry bread, cubed
    fine
1 onion, chopped fine
1½ teaspoons salt

⅓ teaspoon pepper
¾ teaspoon nutmeg
2 tablespoons salad oil
½ cup water
8 onions, peeled
1¼ cups condensed beef
    bouillon
1 teaspoon oregano
¼ teaspoon paprika

Mix first eight ingredients well; let stand a few minutes. Divide
mixture into patties; brown well in oil on both sides. Drain on
brown paper or paper towel. Pour fat from pan; add remaining
ingredients to pan. Return patties to mixture; cover and cook
gently 30 minutes.

MAINE SUPPER

Exchanges per serving: 1 serving = 2 Starch, 1 Fat, 3 Lean Meat
Calories per serving: 325   Yield: 6 servings

1 tablespoon onion,
  chopped
2 tablespoons green
  pepper, chopped
2 tablespoons diet
  margarine
4 cups pork and beans

Nonnutritive sweetener
  equivalent to 1½ cups
  brown sugar
½ cup celery chopped
1 cup Vienna sausages,
  each sliced in half

Brown onion and pepper in margarine. Add pork and beans, sweetener, and celery. Mix together and divide among 6 individual casseroles. Place ⅙ of sausage pieces in each casserole; bake at 350°F until browned.

CHARLOTTE'S CURRIED CHICKEN

Exchanges per serving: ½ cup sauce with chicken over ½ cup
rice = 1 Starch, ⅓ Fruit, 2½ Lean Meat,
⅓ Vegetable

Calories per serving: 256   Yield: 6 servings

1 cup long-grain white rice	1 chicken bouillon cube
1 tablespoon diet margarine	1 teaspoon salt
	1½ teaspoons curry powder
2 chicken breasts (16–18 ounces total) split, boned, and cut into 2″–3″ pieces	½ tablespoon arrowroot
	¾ cup nonfat milk
	1 cup water
1 cup mushrooms, sliced thin	1 cup apples, sliced
	1 teaspoon parsley, chopped fine
½ cup onions, chopped fine	

Cook rice as directed, adding ½ tablespoon margarine. Sauté
chicken, mushrooms, and onions in remaining ½ tablespoon
margarine until chicken is lightly browned on all sides (about
15 minutes). Combine bouillon cube, which has been finely
crushed, salt, curry powder, arrowroot, and some of the milk
to make a smooth paste; then add remaining milk, water, apple, and parsley. Cook until thick and smooth and apple is tender, stirring constantly. Stir chicken into sauce; serve over the
rice.

CHICKEN LIVERS

Exchanges per serving: 1 serving = ¼ Fat, 3 Lean Meat,
1 Vegetable

Calories per serving: 206   Yield: 4 servings

2 onions, sliced thin	1 pound chicken livers
2 stalks celery, sliced thin	½ teaspoon salt
1 tablespoon diet margarine	¼ teaspoon pepper

Sauté onions and celery in margarine until celery is wilted. Remove vegetables, leaving fat in pan. Add chicken livers; turn

heat high; cook, turning once or twice, until done (3–5 minutes). Top with onions and celery. Season with salt and pepper.

CHICKEN SUPERB

Exchanges per serving: 1 serving = ½ Fat, ¼ Fruit, 3 Lean
Meat, ½ Starch

Calories per serving: 260   Yield: 4 servings

¼ cup flour
1 teaspoon salt
⅛ teaspoon pepper
2 chicken breasts, split and skinned
2 tablespoons diet margarine
½ green pepper, chopped fine

¼ cup pimento, diced fine
½ cup mushrooms, cut in quarters
¼ teaspoon ginger
1 cup canned chicken broth
¼ cup orange juice
½ orange, unpeeled and sliced thin

Mix together flour, salt, and half the pepper. Lightly coat chicken with flour mixture. Cook chicken in margarine until golden, using a tightly covered pan. Turn breasts meat side down; add remaining ingredients; cover. Stirring occasionally, simmer gently until tender (about 30 minutes).

BROILED SPRING CHICKEN

Exchanges per serving: 2 ounces = 2 Lean Meat
Calories per serving: 110   Yield: 8 2-ounce servings

2- to 3-pound broiling chicken, dressed, cut into serving pieces

2 tablespoons diet margarine, melted
Dash of seasoned salt
Dash of lemon pepper

Preheat oven to 500°F. Brush chicken with margarine; rub with salt and pepper. Place under broiler; brown evenly; turn and brown other side. Allow 30 minutes or more to cook so the joints are not rare. Baste with pan juices from time to time, adding water if needed.

SAUCES

BERRY SAUCE

Exchanges per serving: 1 tablespoon = None
¼ cup = ½ Fruit
Calories per serving: 5 (per tablespoon)   Yield: 1½ cups

Nonnutritive sweetener
  equivalent to ½ cup sugar
1 teaspoon arrowroot
Dash of salt
½ cup water

1 cup berries (e.g.,
  blueberries, raspberries)
1 tablespoon lemon juice
1 teaspoon lemon rind,
  grated

Combine sweetener, arrowroot, and salt; stir in water. Add berries. Bring to a boil; simmer until clear and thick, about 5 minutes. Remove from heat; add lemon juice and rind. Chill and use over ice creams, custards, plain cakes, waffles, or pancakes.

BARB'S BARBECUE SAUCE

Exchanges per serving: ½ cup = 1 Vegetable
Calories per serving: 30   Yield: 2 cups

½ cup onions, chopped
  fine
⅔ cup tomato paste
1 cup water
1 teaspoon Worcestershire
  sauce
2 teaspoons maple extract
2 tablespoons garlic-
  flavored vinegar

¼ cup catsup (see
  following recipe)
1 teaspoon salt
⅛ teaspoon pepper
¼ teaspoon dried oregano,
  crushed fine
¼ teaspoon dried
  rosemary, crushed fine

Blend all ingredients together in a saucepan; simmer over low heat about 30 minutes, or until onions are well cooked. Use with any broiled meat such as lamb patties, ground beef, beef, pork, or lamb chops.

CATSUP

Exchanges per serving: 1 tablespoon = None
Calories per serving: 6   Yield: 2 cups

4 tomatoes, quartered
⅓ cup green pepper, chopped fine
2 tablespoons red pepper, chopped very fine
½ cup malt vinegar
½ teaspoon salt
Nonnutritive sweetener equivalent to 1 cup sugar
¼ teaspoon cinnamon
⅛ teaspoon allspice
⅛ teaspoon anise seed, crushed fine
¼ teaspoon ground mustard
¼ teaspoon powdered red pepper
¼ teaspoon mace

If using blender, fill ¾ full with first three ingredients; blend about 3–4 seconds at highest speed. If not using blender, mix until pureed. Pour mixture into pan; add vinegar, salt, and sweetener. Tie spices loosely together in a bag of cheesecloth and add. Simmer, uncovered, until reduced by about half. Re move bag of spices.

GRAVY

Exchanges per serving: 1 tablespoon = None
Calories per serving: 4   Yield: 2 cups

1 onion, thinly sliced
2 stalks celery, diced
1¼ cups chicken broth (or condensed beef consommé)
1¼ cups water
¼ teaspoon Gravy Master
1 tablespoon arrowroot

Combine onion, celery, broth, and water in a medium saucepan; cover and boil gently over low heat until onion is transparent. Strain. Reserve vegetables for later use. Return broth to pan. Use a little water, Gravy Master, and arrowroot to make a smooth paste; stir slowly into broth and heat to boiling.

MINT SAUCE

Exchanges per serving: 1 tablespoon = None
Calories per serving: 0   Yield: 1¾ cups

¾ cup vinegar
1 cup water
½ cup mint leaves,
   chopped
¼ cup lemon juice

Nonnutritive sweetener
   equivalent to 1½
   tablespoons sugar
½ teaspoon salt

Heat vinegar and ½ cup water to boiling. Pour over half the mint leaves. Let stand 15 minutes. Strain; add remaining water, lemon juice, sweetener, and salt; chill. Add remaining mint leaves just before serving. Serve with lamb.

SWEET AND TANGY TOMATO SAUCE
FOR SPARERIBS AND LOIN OF PORK

Exchanges per serving: ½ cup = 1 Vegetable
Calories per serving: 28   Yield: 2½ cups

⅓ cup vinegar
Nonnutritive sweetener
   equivalent to 1½ cups
   sugar
2 tablespoons
   Worcestershire sauce

2 tablespoons prepared
   mustard
½ teaspoon Tabasco sauce
¼ cup onion, minced
2 cups tomato sauce

Combine all ingredients in a saucepan; bring to a boil. Use to baste spareribs or loin of pork.

HOT SHOYU (SOY) SAUCE

Exchanges per serving: 2 tablespoons = None
Calories per serving: 8   Yield: 1⅔ cups

1 cup soy sauce
⅔ cup water
Nonnutritive sweetener
  equivalent to ½ cup
  brown sugar

¼ teaspoon instant onion
1 teaspoon arrowroot
  powder

Blend all ingredients; heat to light boil. Serve as dip for shrimp tempura or "pupus," or as sauce for fish or chicken.

BARBECUE SAUCE

Exchanges per serving: 1 tablespoon = None
Calories per serving: 2   Yield: 2 cups

4 tablespoons lemon juice
Dash of red pepper
2 tablespoons cider vinegar
1 cup low-calorie catsup
  (see catsup recipe)
½ cup water
3 tablespoons
  Worcestershire sauce

Dash of lemon pepper
1½ teaspoons mustard
Nonnutritive sweetener
  equivalent to ½ cup
  sugar
½ teaspoon salt

Combine all ingredients; simmer over medium heat about 20–25 minutes.

COLD SHOYU (SOY) SAUCE

Exchanges per serving: 1 tablespoon = None
Calories per serving: 9   Yield: ¾ cup

½ cup soy sauce   2 tablespoons wine vinegar
Nonnutritive sweetener
  equivalent to 3
  tablespoons brown sugar

Blend ingredients well. Serve in small bowls with hot fried foods, cold meat, or fish "pupus."

TOMATO SAUCE

Exchanges per serving: ¼ cup = ½ Vegetable
Calories per serving: 15   Yield: 3 cups

½ onion, chopped fine   ¼ teaspoon basil
1 tablespoon olive oil   Nonnutritive sweetener
½ clove garlic, minced fine   equivalent to ¼ teaspoon
2 cups tomato sauce   sugar
1 cup water   ¼ teaspoon salt

Sauté onion in oil until lightly browned; add garlic and sauté until lightly browned. Stir in remaining ingredients; simmer 1 hour. If using for spaghetti, simmer 5 hours.

GOLDEN SHOYU DIP

Exchanges per serving: 1 tablespoon = 1½ Fat
Calories per serving: 78   Yield: 1¼ cups

1 cup safflower   ½ teaspoon instant onion
  mayonnaise   ¼ teaspoon arrowroot
¼ cup soy sauce

Blend all ingredients until smooth; cook until consistency desired; chill. Restir before serving as dip for all fish "pupus" or with grilled or fried fish.

SWEET AND SOUR MARINADE
(For shish kabobs and brochettes)

Exchanges per serving: ½ cup = ½ Fruit
Calories per serving: 28   Yield: 2 cups

1 cup soy sauce
½ cup vinegar
½ cup unsweetened
    pineapple juice

Nonnutritive sweetener
    equivalent to 1½ cups
    sugar
½ teaspoon salt
½ teaspoon garlic powder

Combine all ingredients; bring to a boil. Marinate beef or lamb
cubes in mixture for at least four hours in the refrigerator. Also
useful for basting meat while cooking.

TANGY TONGUE SAUCE

Exchanges per serving: ¼ cup = ½ Fat, ½ Fruit
Calories per serving: 56   Yield: 3¼ cups

¼ cup diet margarine
2 tablespoons arrowroot
1½ cups unsweetened
    apple juice
¾ cup beer

2 tablespoons white
    vinegar
Nonnutritive sweetener
    equivalent to 2
    tablespoons brown sugar
½ cup raisins

Melt margarine and stir in arrowroot; gradually add apple juice
and beer, stirring constantly. Add remaining ingredients; cook
over low heat, stirring, until sauce is smooth and slightly thickened. Serve over hot or cold tongue.

TARTAR SAUCE

Exchanges per serving: 2 tablespoons = 1 Fat
Calories per serving: 45   Yield: ½ cup

¼ cup imitation
mayonnaise
2 tablespoons dill pickle,
chopped
1 tablespoon diet
margarine

2 tablespoons parsley,
minced
1 teaspoon lemon juice
¼ teaspoon salt

Mix all ingredients together, chill before serving. Store in refrigerator.

CELERY AND TOMATO SAUCE

Exchanges per serving: ½ cup = ¼ Fat, ½ Vegetable
Calories per serving: 32   Yield: 2 cups

1 tablespoon green pepper,
minced fine
2 tablespoons dried onion
1 cup celery, sliced thin
1 tablespoon diet
margarine
1 scant cup tomato sauce

½ teaspoon sesame seeds,
crushed fine
¼ teaspoon lemon pepper
Dash of salt
Dash of black pepper
¼ teaspoon garlic salt

Sauté pepper, onion, and celery in margarine until golden and wilted. Add remaining ingredients; boil gently about 30 minutes. Serve over fish or meat.

SPAGHETTI SAUCE

Exchanges per serving: 1 cup = 1 Vegetable
Calories per serving: 30 (sauce only)   Yield: 10 cups

½ cup celery, chopped fine	½ teaspoon marjoram
1½ cups onion, chopped fine	⅛ teaspoon celery salt
	Dash of garlic salt
1 tablespoon diet margarine	¼ teaspoon rosemary
	1 teaspoon oregano
8 cups tomatoes	½ teaspoon basil
1 cup tomato sauce	¼ teaspoon salt
½ teaspoon thyme	Dash of pepper

Sauté celery and onion in margarine until golden and wilted; add remaining ingredients. Cover and bring to a boil. Uncover and boil gently until sauce is thick. Use for noodles, spaghetti, macaroni, or meat.

RAISIN SAUCE

Exchanges per serving: 2 tablespoons = ½ Fruit
Calories per serving: 24   Yield: 1½ cups

Nonnutritive sweetener equivalent to ¾ cup brown sugar	1½ cups broth (preferably tongue)
	¼ cup vinegar
1½ tablespoons arrowroot	½ cup golden raisins
	1 lemon, sliced thin

Mix sweetener and arrowroot in top of double boiler; add broth gradually, stirring constantly. Add remaining ingredients. Cook until raisins are plump and mixture thick, stirring constantly. Serve hot with ham or tongue.

CHINESE MUSTARD

Exchanges per serving: 1 tablespoon = ¼ Fat
Calories per serving: 16   Yield: ½ cup

⅓ cup dry mustard
1 tablespoon safflower oil
Nonnutritive sweetener
   equivalent to 1 teaspoon
   sugar

½ teaspoon seasoned salt
2 teaspoons flat beer or
   wine

Mix all ingredients until smooth; serve in small dipping bowl.

APPLE-CRANBERRY RELISH

Exchanges per serving: ¼ cup = ¼ Fat, ¾ Fruit
Calories per serving: 74   Yield: 2 cups

½ cup apples, diced
2 cups fresh cranberries,
   chopped fine
¼ cup white raisins,
   chopped fine

¼ cup walnuts, chopped
   fine
Nonnutritive sweetener
   equivalent to 1 cup sugar
½ teaspoon lemon juice

Combine all ingredients, mixing well. Chill overnight in refrigerator.

LOW-CALORIE TOPPING WHIP

Exchanges per serving: ¼ cup = None
Calories per serving: 9   Yield: 3½ cups

½ cup nonfat dry milk
½ cup ice water
2 tablespoons fresh lemon
   juice

Nonnutritive sweetener
   equivalent to ¼ cup
   sugar

Place bowl and beaters in refrigerator for about two hours. Mix nonfat milk powder and ice water in chilled bowl; beat with mixer until soft peaks form. Add juice and sweetener; beat again until mixture forms stiff peaks.

CUSTARD SAUCE FOR SHORTCAKE
(High cholesterol)

Exchanges per serving: 1 tablespoon = None
Calories per serving: 9   Yield: 2½ cups

2 cups nonfat milk	½ tablespoon arrowroot
2 eggs	¼ teaspoon salt
Nonnutritive sweetener	1 teaspoon vanilla extract
equivalent to 1½ cups	1 teaspoon almond extract
sugar	

Scald milk in saucepan. Beat eggs, sweetener, arrowroot, and salt in small bowl; gradually add scalded milk. Return mixture to saucepan; cook over low heat, stirring constantly, until mixture coats a spoon and is slightly thickened. Remove from heat; beat in vanilla and almond extracts. Chill until ready to use.

CHERRY GLAZE

Exchanges per serving: ½ cup = ⅓ Fruit
Calories per serving: 37   Yield: 3 cups

2 cups sour red cherries,	1 teaspoon arrowroot
water-packed, pitted;	1 tablespoon lemon juice
reserve liquid	¼ teaspoon almond extract
Nonnutritive sweetener	Drop of red vegetable food
equivalent to 2	coloring (optional)
tablespoons sugar	

Mix ½ cup liquid from cherries with sweetener and arrowroot; stir to make smooth paste. Cook, stirring constantly, until thick and smooth. Add cherries, lemon juice, almond extract, and coloring, if desired. Allow to cool at room temperature. May be used over dietetic ice cream and on pineapple cheese pie, among other desserts.

LEMON SAUCE

Exchanges per serving: 5 tablespoons = ½ Fat

Calories per serving: 23   Yield: 1 cup

¾ tablespoon arrowroot
Nonnutritive sweetener
 equivalent to ½ cup
 sugar
⅛ teaspoon salt
1 cup boiling water
2 tablespoons diet
 margarine

1½ tablespoons lemon
 juice
1½ teaspoons lemon rind,
 grated fine
Dash of anise seed,
 crushed fine
Dash of nutmeg
Dash of cloves

Combine arrowroot, sweetener, and salt in saucepan; add boiling water slowly, stirring to avoid lumps. Simmer and stir until thick; remove from heat. Stir in margarine and remaining ingredients. Use for cake fillings and over bread puddings and custards.

CUSTARD SAUCE

Exchanges per serving: ½ cup = ¾ Medium-Fat Meat,
                                        ⅓ Nonfat Milk

Calories per serving: 62   Yield: 4 servings

1 whole egg plus 2 egg
 yolks
Nonnutritive sweetener
 equivalent to 3
 tablespoons sugar

⅛ teaspoon salt
1½ cups nonfat milk
1 teaspoon vanilla extract

Beat 1 egg and 2 yolks together in saucepan (reserve 2 extra whites, covered, in refrigerator, for use another time). Blend in sweetener and salt; gradually stir in nonfat milk. Place over low heat, stirring constantly, until mixture thickens slightly and coats a metal spoon. Remove from heat; stir in vanilla; chill. (Sauce will thicken more during chilling.)

POLLY'S CUSTARD SAUCE

Exchanges per serving: ½ cup = ½ Medium-Fat Meat,
                                             ½ Nonfat Milk

Calories per serving: 82   Yield: 3½ cups

3 cups nonfat milk
Nonnutritive sweetener
  equivalent to ½ cup
  sugar

1 tablespoon arrowroot
½ cup egg yolks
1 teaspoon almond extract

Combine nonfat milk and sweetener in top of double boiler;
heat. Mix arrowroot and egg yolks; beat well. Add small
amount of hot mixture to egg mixture; blend. Gradually blend
egg mixture into milk and cook over simmering water, stirring
constantly, until mixture is slightly thickened (about 15 minutes). Remove from heat; pour at once into heatproof bowl. Stir
in almond extract; place in refrigerator to chill. (Sauce will
thicken more as it chills.)

ORANGE SAUCE

Exchanges per serving: ¼ cup = ½ Fruit
Calories per serving: 22   Yield: 2 cups

Nonnutritive sweetener
  equivalent to 1 cup sugar
¼ teaspoon salt
1 tablespoon arrowroot
1 cup orange juice
¼ cup lemon juice
¾ cup boiling water

1 tablespoon diet
  margarine
1 teaspoon grated orange
  peel
1 teaspoon grated lemon
  peel

Combine sweetener, salt, and arrowroot; stir in orange and
lemon juices, and boiling water. Boil 1 minute, stirring constantly. Remove from heat; stir in margarine and orange and
lemon peels. Serve over hot cake or pudding.

SAUCE ROYALE

Exchanges per serving: ½ cup = ½ Fat
Calories per serving: 23   Yield: 4 servings

1 tablespoon arrowroot	Dash of salt
4 tablespoons cold water	Nonnutritive sweetener
½ teaspoon nutmeg	equivalent to 1 cup sugar
½ teaspoon cinnamon	2 tablespoons diet
⅛ teaspoon allspice	margarine
2 cups boiling water	

Dissolve arrowroot in cold water; add spices. Add mixture to boiling water. Stir, bring to simmer; add salt, sweetener, and margarine. Use hot for custards.

SAUCE CHERRIE

Exchanges per serving: ½ cup = 1 Fruit
Calories per serving: 52   Yield: 2 cups

1 teaspoon arrowroot	1 teaspoon vanilla extract
2 cups water-packed	Nonnutritive sweetener
cherries, undrained	equivalent to ½ cup
½ teaspoon almond extract	sugar

Combine arrowroot and cherries; bring to boil and simmer 5–6 minutes. Remove from heat; add extracts and sweetener. Serve slightly warm over dietetic ice cream, custards, and the like.

CHOCOLATE SAUCE

Exchanges per serving: 1 tablespoon = 2 Fat
Calories per serving: 93   Yield: 1 cup

8 ounces unsweetened	Nonnutritive sweetener
chocolate	equivalent to ¼ cup sugar
¼ cup water	½ cup nondairy whipped
	topping

Combine chocolate, water, and sweetener. Melt over hot water in double boiler. Stir until smooth; remove from heat; cool. Blend in whipped topping. Serve either hot or cold.

CITRUS FRUIT SAUCE

Exchanges per serving: ¼ cup = ½ Fat
Calories per serving: 31   Yield: 1 cup

Nonnutritive sweetener
  equivalent to ½ cup
  sugar
2 teaspoons arrowroot
⅛ teaspoon salt
1 cup boiling water
2 tablespoons diet
  margarine, melted

1½ tablespoons fruit juice
  (grapefruit, lemon, or
  orange)
1½ teaspoons grated fruit
  rind
Dash of nutmeg

Combine sweetener, arrowroot, and salt in a saucepan. Stir in boiling water until smooth; stir and simmer until clear and thick. Stir in remaining ingredients.

HAWAIIAN CURRY SAUCE

Exchanges per serving: ½ cup = 3 Fat, ½ Fruit, ½ Skim Milk
Calories per serving: 212 (sauce only)   Yield: 2 cups

¼ cup safflower oil
1 onion, minced
2 apples, peeled and diced
2½ teaspoons arrowroot
2 cups nonfat milk or
  coconut milk

1 teaspoon garlic salt
1 teaspoon salt
1 teaspoon ground ginger
3 tablespoons soy sauce
1–3 teaspoons curry
  powder (to taste)

Heat oil. Add onion and apples; cover and cook 10 minutes, stirring occasionally. Add arrowroot and stir until smooth; add nonfat milk or coconut milk with remaining ingredients, stirring constantly until mixture thickens and boils. Reduce heat to very low; cover and cook 20 minutes. Mix sauce with 2 cups cooked seafood, chicken, or meat and serve on steamed rice, or as called for in recipe.

MAPLE-FLAVORED SAUCE

Exchanges per serving: ¼ cup = Fat, ⅓ Skim Milk
Calories per serving: 53   Yield: 1¾ cups

¼ cup diet margarine
1 tablespoon arrowroot
Nonnutritive sweetener
  equivalent to 1 cup sugar
½ cup water

1 cup nonfat evaporated
  milk
1½ teaspoons maple
  flavoring

Melt margarine. Blend in arrowroot; add sweetener, water, and milk. Cook over medium heat, stirring constantly until thick. Remove from heat; add maple flavoring and chill.

VEGETABLES

See Packaged Food tables for additional suggestions.

JUICES

Tomato Juice, 6 ounces.........................35 calories
Vegetable Cocktail Juice, 6 ounces ....35 calories

EGGPLANT, PEPPER, AND MUSHROOMS

Exchanges per serving: 1 cup = 1½ Fat, 1 Vegetable
Calories per serving: 90   Yield: 12 cups

1 eggplant, cut and diced into squares (4 cups)	2 cups tomatoes, peeled and diced
⅓ cup oil	1 clove garlic, minced very fine
½ cup water	
2 large green peppers, cored and diced	1 teaspoon salt
1 cup sliced mushrooms, drained	Nonnutritive sweetener equivalent to 1 teaspoon sugar
	½ teaspoon pepper

Place squares of eggplant (unpeeled) into frying pan with 3 tablespoons heated oil. Sauté over medium heat 2 minutes, turning often. Add 2 tablespoons water; cover and cook, adding water, 2 tablespoons at a time, as it is absorbed. Turn eggplant occasionally until tender (about 10 minutes). Remove from pan into bowl. Add balance of oil to pan; sauté peppers about 10 minutes; add mushrooms and heat until soft; add to eggplant. Add remaining ingredients to pan; simmer until mixture becomes a thick sauce; pour over eggplant. Mix lightly.

EGGPLANT DELIGHT

Exchanges per serving: 1 cup = ⅓ Fat, 1½ Vegetable
Calories per serving: 48   Yield: 6 cups

1 onion, sliced thick	3 cups eggplant, peeled,
¼ green pepper, chopped	cubed
fine	2 cups tomatoes
2 tablespoons diet	½ teaspoon salt
margarine	⅛ teaspoon pepper

Sauté onion and pepper in margarine in medium skillet, tightly
covered, until soft. Add eggplant cubes, tomatoes, salt, and pepper, cover. Simmer until eggplant is tender (about 10 minutes).

DORIS'S CREAMED MUSHROOMS

Exchanges per serving: ½ cup = ½ Fat, ½ Vegetable
Calories per serving: 40   Yield: 6 cups

1 envelope dry cream of	3 tablespoons diet
mushroom soup mix	margarine
2 cups water	1 tablespoon lemon juice
4 cups fresh mushrooms	Dash of salt
	Dash of pepper

Add soup mix to water; boil gently, stirring now and then, for
about 10 minutes. Sauté mushrooms in margarine in large skillet until browned on all sides. Pour soup and lemon juice over
mushrooms. Season.

CREAMED SPINACH

Exchanges per serving: ⅔ cup = ⅓ Fat, 1 Vegetable,
⅟₄ Skim Milk

Calories per serving: 65   Yield: 2 cups

1 clove garlic, minced fine	½ teaspoon salt
1 tablespoon diet margarine	⅛ teaspoon pepper
	½ teaspoon arrowroot
1¼ cups frozen spinach, chopped	½ cup nonfat milk

Sauté garlic in margarine until brown; discard garlic. Add spinach, which has been thoroughly thawed, salt, and pepper; separate spinach with a fork. Cover tightly. Cook over low heat until spinach is tender and liquid has evaporated (about 4–5 minutes). Form a smooth paste of arrowroot and milk; add to cooked spinach. Heat, stirring constantly, until thick and smooth.

GOURMET SPINACH

Exchanges per serving: Scant ½ cup = 1 Fat, 1 Vegetable
Calories per serving: 64   Yield: 2¾ cups

1 cup mushrooms, thinly sliced	1¼ cups frozen spinach, chopped
1 onion chopped fine	½ cup imitation sour cream or sour half-and-half
1 clove garlic, minced	
1 tablespoon diet margarine	1 teaspoon salt
	⅛ teaspoon pepper

Sauté mushrooms, onion, and garlic in margarine until onion is golden. Place spinach on top of mushroom mixture; cover, stirring now and then. Cook until spinach is heated through (8–9 minutes). Stir in sour cream, salt, and pepper.

GREEN BEAN SPECIAL

Exchanges per serving: ¾ cup = 1 Vegetable
Calories per serving: 18   Yield: 4½ cups

1 wafer-thin strip bacon	2½ cups green beans
1 clove garlic, minced fine	1¼ teaspoons salt
¼ cup onion, chopped fine	⅛ teaspoon pepper
2 tablespoons green pepper, chopped fine	½ teaspoon oregano
1 cup tomatoes, chopped	⅓ cup water

Cook, drain, and crumble wafer-thin strip of bacon. Pour out all fat, leaving a light coating in pan. Sauté garlic, onion, and pepper until onion is golden. Stir in bacon and remaining ingredients; cover. Cook gently until beans are tender (about 15 minutes).

GREEN BEANS DE LUXE

Exchanges per serving: ¾ cup = ½ Fat, 1 Vegetable
Calories per serving: 38   Yield: 4½ cups

4 cups canned green beans, undrained	2 tablespoons diet margarine
¼ cup mint flakes, dried	Dash of salt
Nonnutritive sweetener equivalent to 1 tablespoon sugar	Dash of pepper

Heat beans and mint flakes with sweetener to boiling point; drain. Stir in remaining ingredients.

ASPARAGUS WITH HERBS

Exchanges per serving: 1 serving = ⅓ Fat, ½ Vegetable
Calories per serving: 32   Yield: 3 servings

1 tablespoon diet margarine	2 tablespoons chives, chopped
½ teaspoon salt	1¼ cups asparagus
¼ cup water	Dash of seasoned salt
	Dash of pepper

Place margarine, salt, water, and chives in skillet; cover tightly.
Bring to boil. Add asparagus; cover and boil gently until asparagus is tender. Sprinkle with seasoned salt and pepper.

PEAS AND LETTUCE

Exchanges per serving: 1 serving = 1 Fat, ½ Starch,
                    ¼ Vegetable
Calories per serving: 90   Yield: 4 servings

1¼ cups frozen peas	4 tablespoons diet margarine (or omit margarine and delete fat exchange)
1 cup lettuce, coarsely torn	

Cook peas in boiling salted water until tender (5–6 minutes);
add lettuce and simmer until wilted and transparent. Drain.
Toss with margarine.

BEETS WILLIAM-STYLE

Exchanges per serving: 1 serving = ½ Vegetable
Calories per serving: 30   Yield: 4 servings

Nonnutritive sweetener   ½ teaspoon pepper
  equivalent to 2   ¾ teaspoon arrowroot
  tablespoons sugar   2 cups sliced beets
½ teaspoon salt   2 tablespoons lemon juice

Mix sweetener, salt, pepper, and arrowroot. Drain liquid from
beets, saving ⅓ cup. Stir the ⅓ cup liquid with lemon juice and
drained beets into sweetened mixture. Boil until sauce thickens
and beets are heated, stirring constantly.

TOMATOES WITH CHEESE TOPPING

Exchanges per serving: 1 serving = ¼ High-Fat Meat,
                                    1 Vegetable
Calories per serving: 45   Yield: 4 servings

2 tomatoes, peeled and   2 tablespoons seasoned
  halved   dried bread crumbs
½ teaspoon thyme   ½ teaspoon salt
2 tablespoons American   ⅛ teaspoon pepper
  cheese, finely grated

Preheat oven to 375°F. Place tomatoes, cut side up, in baking
pan; top each half with a mixture of remaining ingredients.
Bake until tomatoes are tender and cheese melts (about 20 minutes). Put baking pan under broiler for the last minute or so, to
brown tops.

CELERY AND CARROTS
(WITH HORSERADISH)

Exchanges per serving: 1 serving = ⅓ Fat, ½ Vegetable
Calories per serving: 32   Yield: 6 servings

2 cups carrots, cut into ½″
  slices
⅔ cup celery, cut into ½″
  pieces
½ cup water

1½ teaspoons prepared
  horseradish
½ teaspoon salt
2 tablespoons diet
  margarine

Scrape carrots before slicing; remove any strings from celery
and slice. Place carrots and celery in saucepan with water,
horseradish, and salt; cover tightly and boil until tender (about
20 minutes). Drain and add margarine.

SWEET CARROTS

Exchanges per serving: ⅔ cup = ½ Fat, 1 Vegetable
Calories per serving: 50   Yield: 2 cups

1 tablespoon diet
  margarine
2 tablespoons water
½ teaspoon salt
⅛ teaspoon pepper

Nonnutritive sweetener
  equivalent to ½ teaspoon
  sugar
2 tablespoons parsley,
  snipped fine
2 cups carrots, scraped and
  sliced thin

Melt margarine; add remaining ingredients. Cover; simmer
gently about 10 minutes, stirring occasionally.

GINGERED CARROTS

Exchanges per serving: ½ cup = ½ Fat, ½ Vegetable
Calories per serving: 36   Yield: 2½ cups

2 cups carrots, cut julienne
½ cup water
½ teaspoon Mei Yen
   seasoning
½ teaspoon ginger

Nonnutritive sweetener
   equivalent to ½ teaspoon
   sugar
2 tablespoons diet
   margarine

Cook carrots in water seasoned with Mei Yen powder; add ginger and sweetener; when carrots are tender, add margarine. Continue to cook 3–4 minutes, stirring gently.

CARROTS WITH ORANGE

Exchanges per serving: ½ cup = ⅓ Fat, ½ Vegetable
Calories per serving: 37   Yield: 6 servings

3 teaspoons salt
Water to cover carrots
3 cups carrots, scraped and
   thinly sliced

Nonnutritive sweetener
   equivalent to 1
   tablespoon sugar
2 tablespoons diet
   margarine
1 orange, cut into sections

Place 2 teaspoons salt in water; gently boil carrots until tender. Add remaining salt, sweetener, margarine, and oranges. Heat slowly and gently.

DELIGHTFUL CARROTS

Exchanges per serving: 1 serving = 1 Fat, 1 Vegetable
Calories per serving: 70   Yield: 4 servings

6 carrots, peeled and cut
   into 3″ strips
4 tablespoons diet
   margarine

1 tablespoon lemon juice
⅛ teaspoon celery seed
½ teaspoon salt
2 tablespoons water

Preheat oven to 350°F. Arrange carrots in small baking dish. Melt margarine and combine with remaining ingredients. Pour over carrots. Cover and bake about 45 minutes, or until carrots are tender.

CARROTS WITH CHEESE

Exchanges per serving: 1 cup = 2 Lean Meat, 1 Vegetable
Calories per serving: 135   Yield: 2 cups

2 cups carrots, sliced	⅛ teaspoon salt
½ cup cheese, grated—	⅛ teaspoon pepper
Neufchâtel or Parmesan	1 tablespoon parsley flakes

Boil carrots gently in water to cover about 5 minutes; turn off heat and drain thoroughly. Return to saucepan; sprinkle with cheese, letting carrots stay over low heat until cheese melts. Sprinkle with salt and pepper and top with parsley.

SWEET AND SOUR RED CABBAGE

Exchanges per serving: 1 serving = ½ Fruit, 1 Vegetable
Calories per serving: 45   Yield: 8 servings

1 small head red cabbage	3 tablespoons fructose
2 teaspoons cornstarch	¼ teaspoon salt
½ cup water	½ teaspoon caraway seeds
½ cup cider vinegar	

Shred cabbage; steam over rapidly boiling water 10 minutes, or until crisp-tender. Remove from heat; drain thoroughly. Dissolve cornstarch in water; add remaining ingredients; cook over medium heat until slightly thickened. Put cooked cabbage in large mixing bowl; add sauce and mix well. Use this dish with either hot or cold meat.

NOTE: This recipe is provided through the courtesy of Sweet Lite Fructose.

PINEAPPLE SWEET POTATOES

Exchanges per serving: ½ cup (approximately 5 ounces) =
1 Starch, ¼ Fat, ½ Fruit

Calories per serving: 122   Yield: 8 servings

24 ounces (1½ lbs.) sweet
potatoes
1½ teaspoons salt
⅛ teaspoon pepper

2 cups artificially
sweetened pineapple
tidbits
2 tablespoons diet
margarine

Boil potatoes until tender; peel; cool slightly. Mash until smooth; stir in remaining ingredients, including syrup from pineapple tidbits. Return to stove and reheat.

BAKED POTATOES, STUFFED

Exchanges per serving: 1 potato = 1⅓ Starch, 1½ Fat
Calories per serving: 150   Yield: 8 servings

8 potatoes (4 ounces each)
1 tablespoon oil
1½ cups sour half-and-half
1½ teaspoons salt

⅛ teaspoon pepper
2 tablespoons chives,
snipped

Preheat oven to 450°F. Prick skins of potatoes with fork; lightly oil your hands and rub oil onto the potatoes. Place potatoes in oven and bake until done (about 35–40 minutes). Reduce heat to 325°F. Remove potatoes from oven; cut a thin slice from each and hollow out, being careful to leave shell intact. Mash centers in mixer with sour half-and-half, salt, pepper, and chives; refill shells, heaping high. Bake on aluminum foil until heated through and top is lightly browned (about ½ hour).

ANNE'S STUFFED BAKED POTATOES WITH CHEESE

Exchanges per serving: 1 potato = 1 Starch, 1 Fat,
                                                    1 High-Fat Meat
Calories per serving: 175   Yield: 8 servings

8 potatoes (4 ounces each)	Dash of pepper
5 tablespoons diet margarine	1 cup cheese, finely grated—mild cheddar,
½ cup skim milk	American, or Neufchâtel
Dash of salt	

Preheat oven to 400°F. Bake potatoes until done (approximately
1 hour). While hot, cut tops off and scoop insides into mixing
bowl (keeping the 8 shells intact). Add margarine and skim
milk; beat until smooth. Add remaining ingredients and continue beating until mixed thoroughly. Refill potato shells, place
on baking pan for 20 minutes, then under broiler until deli-
cately browned.

MARGE'S STUFFED POTATOES

Exchanges per serving: 1 potato = 1⅓ Starch, 1 Fat
Calories per serving: 165   Yield: 6 servings

6 potatoes (4 ounces each)	3½ tablespoons Parmesan cheese, grated
1 teaspoon salt	
1 tablespoon chives, finely chopped	½ teaspoon pepper
2 tablespoons bacon bits	1 tablespoon imitation sour cream or sour half-
½ cup diet margarine	and-half
	Dash of paprika

Preheat oven to 400°F. Grease potatoes using Pam or similar
coating, then bake until soft. Cut in half lengthwise; spoon out
centers into mixing bowl while hot, saving skins. Add remaining ingredients except paprika; mix about 3 minutes at medium
speed of electric mixer. Place mixture in potato skins. Sprinkle
lightly with paprika and brown in oven about 4 minutes.

POLLY'S CREAMED POTATOES

Exchanges per serving: ¾ cup = 1½ Starch, ⅓ Skim Milk,
⅓ Fat, ¼ Vegetable

Calories per serving: 120   Yield: 8 servings

8 potatoes (4 ounces each), peeled and cubed
1 onion, thinly sliced
1 cup celery, thinly sliced
¾ tablespoon chervil
2 teaspoons salt
⅛ teaspoon pepper

2½ cups nonfat milk
2 tablespoons diet margarine
2 tablespoons water
1½ teaspoons arrowroot
2 tablespoons dried parsley

Mix all ingredients except water, arrowroot, and parsley in saucepan; cook until potatoes are tender (20–25 minutes). Mix water and arrowroot to make a thin paste; stir into potatoes. Cover and cook until thick and smooth, stirring occasionally. Garnish with parsley.

SUPER RICE

Exchanges per serving: Generous ½ cup = 1½ Starch, ¾ Fat
Calories per serving: 145   Yield: 8 servings

1 cup white rice
¼ teaspoon lemon juice
1 cup + 2 tablespoons frozen peas

Nonnutritive sweetener equivalent to 1 tablespoon sugar
1 onion, diced fine
2 tablespoons salad oil
½ teaspoon parsley flakes

Cook rice according to directions on package, but substitute lemon juice for butter. Cook peas; add sweetener. Sauté onion in oil until wilted and golden. Add peas and onion to rice. Garnish with parsley.

BREADS

EASY RAISIN BREAD

Exchanges per serving: 1 slice = 1 Starch
Calories per serving: 94   Yield: 15 slices

- ½ cup quick-cooking oatmeal
- 1 teaspoon baking powder
- 2 cups biscuit mix
- ¼ teaspoon salt
- ½ cup white raisins
- Nonnutritive sweetener equivalent to ¾ cup + 1 tablespoon sugar
- 1 egg, well beaten
- 1¼ cups nonfat milk

Preheat oven to 350°F. Combine dry ingredients; mix remaining ingredients and add to dry ingredients; blend well. Pour into well-greased 1-quart round casserole. Bake until done (about one hour). Cool ten minutes before turning out on rack.

RAISIN BREAD

Exchanges per serving: 1½″ slice = 1 Starch, ½ Fat, ½ Fruit
Calories per serving: 145   Yield: 16 servings

- 3 cups flour
- 3½ teaspoons baking powder
- Nonnutritive sweetener equivalent to ¾ cup sugar
- 1½ teaspoons salt
- ⅓ cup diet margarine
- 1 teaspoon orange peel, grated
- 2 eggs
- 1 cup nonfat milk
- 1 cup white raisins, chopped
- ½ cup nuts, chopped fine

Preheat oven to 350°F. Sift dry ingredients; add margarine, orange peel, eggs, and nonfat milk. Mix until blended; stir in raisins and nuts. Place in well-greased 9″ × 5″ × 3″ loaf pan. Bake 1 hour and 15 minutes or until loaf tests done. Remove from pan; cool and store 12 hours before slicing.

BARBARA'S BANANA BREAD

Exchanges per serving: ¾″ slice = 1 Starch, ⅓ Fat, ¼ Fruit
Calories per serving: 110   Yield: 12 slices

¼ teaspoon baking soda
½ teaspoon salt
1¾ cups flour
2 teaspoons baking
  powder
Nonnutritive granulated
  sweetener equivalent to 1
  cup sugar
¼ cup diet margarine,
  melted
1 egg, well beaten
1 teaspoon almond extract
2 bananas, well mashed

Preheat oven to 350°F. Sift dry ingredients together. Combine margarine, egg, and almond extract; add to first mixture, stirring until flour is moistened. Fold in mashed bananas. Turn into 9″ well-greased loaf pan. Bake until done (about 1 hour).

SHORTBREAD

Exchanges per serving: 1″ × 3″ piece = ¼ Starch, ½ Fat, ⅓ Fruit
Calories per serving: 69   Yield: 36 servings

½ cup diet margarine
Nonnutritive sweetener
  equivalent to 1½ cups
  brown sugar
1 cup plus 2 tablespoons
  flour, sifted
2 eggs
1 teaspoon vanilla extract
1 teaspoon orange peel,
  grated
½ teaspoon salt
1 teaspoon baking powder
1½ cups white raisins,
  chopped
1 cup nuts, chopped fine

Preheat oven to 375°F. Mix margarine, half the sweetener, and 1 cup flour together to fine crumbs; press firmly in the bottom of a 13″ × 9″ × 2″ pan. Bake 10 minutes. Meanwhile, beat eggs until fluffy; beat in remaining sweetener, vanilla, and orange peel. Add remaining flour, salt, and baking powder; mix well. Stir in raisins and nuts; place mixture over crust, which has been slightly cooled. Place entire mixture in oven; bake another 30 minutes. Cool slightly before cutting.

"SEEDED" BREAD

Exchanges per serving: 1 slice = 1 Starch, ⅓ Fat
Calories per serving: 93   Yield: 1 slice

1 slice bread	½ teaspoon poppy seeds
1 teaspoon diet margarine	¼ teaspoon sesame seeds
¼ teaspoon celery seeds	Dash of garlic salt

Spread bread with margarine. Sprinkle with combination of seeds, then garlic salt. Place under broiler until edges of bread are brown and margarine melted. Serve hot or cool (at room temperature).

DATE AND NUT BREAD

Exchanges per serving: 1 slice = 1 Starch, 1 Fat, 1 Fruit
Calories per serving: 156   Yield: 2 loaves (16 slices each)

4 cups dates, pitted	½ cup diet margarine, softened
2 cups nuts, coarsely chopped	Nonnutritive sweetener equivalent to 1¼ cups brown sugar, firmly packed
2 cups boiling water	
2¾ cups flour	
1½ teaspoons baking soda	
1 teaspoon salt	2 eggs
	1 teaspoon vanilla extract

Preheat oven to 350°F. Cut dates into small pieces with scissors; add nuts and boiling water. Allow to cool to room temperature (about 45 minutes). Sift flour with baking soda and salt. On high speed of mixer, beat margarine with sweetener, eggs, and vanilla until smooth. Add date mixture; mix well. Add flour mixture; beat with a wooden spoon until well combined. Place in 2 well-greased 9″ × 5″ × 3″ loaf pans. Bake 70 minutes or until tester inserted in center of bread comes out clean. Cool 10 minutes in pan, then on wire rack until room temperature.

PRUNE BREAD

Exchanges per serving: 1 slice = 1 Starch, ½ Fat, ¾ Fruit
Calories per serving: 254   Yield: 2 loaves (12 slices each)

2 cups dried prunes	1 teaspoon salt
1½ cups boiling water	2 teaspoons baking soda
3 cups flour	2 eggs
Nonnutritive sweetener equivalent to 1½ cups sugar	4 tablespoons salad oil

Preheat oven to 325°F. Soak prunes in cold water for two hours. Drain, then pit and chop prunes. Add boiling water; let stand 5 minutes. Sift flour, sweetener, salt, and baking soda; add prune mixture. Beat; beat in eggs, then salad oil. Pour into two greased 8½″ × 4½″ × 2½″ loaf pans and bake for 1 hour. Remove from pans and cool on wire rack.

CORNBREAD

Exchanges per serving: 1 square = 1½ Starch, ½ Fat
Calories per serving: 145   Yield: 9 squares

1¼ cups flour	1 teaspoon salt
¾ cup yellow cornmeal	1 egg
Nonnutritive sweetener equivalent to 2 tablespoons sugar	⅔ cup nonfat milk
	⅓ cup diet margarine, melted
4½ teaspoons baking powder	

Preheat oven to 425°F. Sift first five ingredients into small bowl. Beat egg well; stir in milk and margarine. Pour into flour mixture all at once; stir until flour is just moistened (mixture will be lumpy). Pour into well-greased 8″ square cake pan. Spread evenly; bake until bread comes away from edges of pan (about 30 minutes). Cut into nine equal squares.

DATE BREAD

Exchanges per serving: 1 slice = 1 Starch, ¼ Fat, ½ Fruit
Calories per serving: 98   Yield: 16 slices

3 cups flour, sifted
1½ teaspoons salt
½ teaspoon ground cloves
½ teaspoon nutmeg
4½ teaspoons baking powder
1 teaspoon mace
½ teaspoon allspice

2 dozen dates, chopped well
1 cup nonfat milk
Nonnutritive sweetener equivalent to 1½ cups sugar
2 eggs, well beaten
¼ cup diet margarine, melted

Preheat oven to 350°F. Sift first seven ingredients together. Add dates; mix nonfat milk, sweetener, eggs, and margarine; add to first mixture. Pour into well-greased 9″ × 5″ × 3″ loaf pan. Bake 1 hour and 15 minutes.

BUTTERMILK BISCUITS WITH SEEDS

Exchanges per serving: 1 biscuit = 1½ Fat, 1 Starch
Calories per serving: 150   Yield: 24 biscuits

4 cups flour
4 teaspoons baking powder
½ teaspoon baking soda
2 teaspoons salt

2 tablespoons seeds (e.g., sesame, caraway)
1½ cups buttermilk
⅔ cup safflower oil

Preheat oven to 350°F. Sift flour, baking powder, baking soda, and salt into bowl; add seeds. Add buttermilk to oil but do not stir together; pour all at once over dry ingredients. Mix with fork to make soft dough. Turn dough onto floured board; knead lightly until smooth; flatten slightly. Cover with sheet of waxed paper; roll to a 6″ × 8″ rectangle about ¼″ thick; remove paper. Cut into 2″ squares. Bake until brown.

JOAN'S BISCUITS

Exchanges per serving: 1 biscuit = 1 Starch, ¼ Fat
Calories per serving: 94   Yield: 16 biscuits

2 cups flour
1 teaspoon salt
3 teaspoons baking
  powder

¼ cup diet margarine
¾ cup nonfat milk

Preheat over to 450°F. Sift flour, salt, and baking powder. Cut in margarine until well mixed with first ingredients; add milk. Knead several times; roll out on lightly floured board until about ½″ thick. Cut with biscuit cutter or inverted glass, or drop by spoonfuls. Place on well-greased heavy-duty aluminum foil or cookie sheet. Bake until browned (13–14 minutes).

CORNMEAL BERRY MUFFINS

Exchanges per serving: 1 muffin = 1 Starch, ½ Fat
Calories per serving: 94   Yield: 15 muffins

⅓ cup diet margarine,
  melted
Nonnutritive sweetener
  equivalent to ⅓ cup
  sugar
¼ cup water
2 eggs
1¼ cups cornmeal

¾ cup flour
2½ teaspoons baking
  powder
¼ teaspoon salt
¾ cup nonfat milk
⅔ cup berries (e.g.,
  blueberries, blackberries)

Preheat oven to 400°F. Beat together margarine, sweetener, water, and eggs; stir in cornmeal. Sift flour, baking powder, and salt. Stir ¼ of this into first mixture with ¼ of the milk. Repeat until used. Wash and drain berries; fold gently into batter. Place about 4 tablespoons in each well-greased muffin cup. Bake until brown and separated from edge of cups (about 20 minutes).

BERRY MUFFINS

Exchanges per serving: 1 muffin = 1 Starch
Calories per serving: 104   Yield: 12 muffins

2 cups biscuit mix
Nonnutritive sweetener
  equivalent to ¼ cup + 2
  tablespoons sugar
1 cup unflavored yogurt

1 egg
1 cup berries (e.g.,
  blueberries, blackberries)
2 teaspoons lemon peel,
  grated

Preheat oven to 425°F. Grease a 12-muffin (2½") tin. Combine
mix and sweetener equivalent to ¼ cup sugar in bowl; add yogurt. Add egg; beat with fork until well combined. Fold berries
gently into batter with rubber spatula; place about ¼ cup batter
into each muffin cup. Combine lemon peel and remaining
sweetener and mix well. Sprinkle over batter; bake until golden
brown (20–25 minutes). Serve hot.

SOUR CREAM MUFFINS

Exchanges per serving: 1 muffin = 1 Starch, 1 Fat
Calories per serving: 151   Yield: 8 muffins

¼ cup diet margarine
¾ cup imitation sour
  cream or sour half-and-
  half
1⅓ cups all-purpose flour,
  sifted

Nonnutritive sweetener
  equivalent to ½ cup
  sugar
½ teaspoon baking soda
¼ teaspoon salt
Dash of nutmeg
1 egg, beaten

Preheat oven to 450°F. Cream margarine; add sour cream; mix
well. Sift dry ingredients. Add alternatively with egg to first
mixture. Spoon into greased muffin tins; bake for 15 minutes.

MARY C'S MUFFINS

Exchanges per serving: 1 muffin = 1 Starch, ½ Fat
Calories per serving: 115   Yield: 24 muffins

½ cup diet margarine	4 cups flour
Nonnutritive sweetener equivalent to ¾ cup sugar	6 teaspoons baking powder
	2 teaspoons salt
3 eggs	1½ cups nonfat milk

Preheat oven to 400°F. Cream together margarine and sweetener. Beat eggs and add. Sift flour, baking powder, and salt together; add alternately with nonfat milk to creamed mixture. Fill well-greased muffin pans ⅔ full. Bake 45 minutes. Serve hot.

LEMON MUFFINS

Exchanges per serving: 1 muffin = 1 Starch, 1¼ Fat
Calories per serving: 149   Yield: 12 muffins

2 cups all-purpose flour, sifted	½ teaspoon salt
	⅔ cup nonfat milk
Nonnutritive sweetener equivalent to ½ cup sugar	⅓ cup lemon juice
	1 teaspoon lemon rind, grated
3 teaspoons baking powder	⅓ cup salad oil
	1 egg, slightly beaten

Preheat oven to 400°F. Sift flour, sweetener, baking powder, and salt into a large bowl. Combine nonfat milk, lemon juice, lemon rind, oil, and egg; beat with a fork to mix well. Pour into dry ingredients; stir quickly with fork (do not beat—batter will be lumpy). Fill each well-greased muffin cup slightly more than half full. Bake 20–25 minutes, until golden (or until cake tester comes out clean). Remove from oven, loosen edges of muffins with spatula, and turn out.

PANCAKES

Exchanges per serving: 1 pancake = 1 Starch
Calories per serving: 90   Yield: ten 4″ pancakes

1¼ cups flour	¾ teaspoon salt
2½ teaspoons baking powder	1 egg
	1¼ cups nonfat milk
Nonnutritive sweetener equivalent to 2 tablespoons sugar	2 tablespoons diet margarine, melted

Mix and sift flour, baking powder, sweetener, and salt in medium bowl. In another bowl beat egg; stir in nonfat milk and margarine; stir into flour mixture until dry ingredients are moist. Heat pan until water dropped on it "jumps" up and down. For each pancake, put about 3 tablespoons of mixture in pan; cook over low heat until bubbles appear on top and under-side is nicely browned. Turn with spatula and brown other side.

WAFFLES

Exchanges per serving: 1 waffle = 1 Starch, ½ Fat
Calories per serving: 102   Yield: ten 4″ waffles

1½ cups flour	Nonnutritive sweetener equivalent to ¼ cup sugar
2 teaspoons baking powder	
½ teaspoon salt	3 tablespoons diet margarine, melted
2 eggs	
1¼ cups nonfat milk	

Heat waffle iron. Sift dry ingredients into bowl. In another bowl, beat eggs, nonfat milk, sweetener, and margarine. Stir mixtures together until flour is moist and batter nearly smooth. Allow 4 tablespoons of batter for each 4″ waffle.

AUNT JEANNE'S COFFEE CAKE

Exchanges per serving: 1 serving = 1½ Starch, 1 Fat
Calories per serving: 170   Yield: 8 servings

2 cups flour
3 teaspoons baking
  powder
¼ teaspoon salt
⅓ cup diet margarine,
  softened
¾ cup nonfat milk
3 drops yellow food
  coloring

Nonnutritive sweetener
  equivalent to ¾ cup
  sugar
1 egg
½ teaspoon cinnamon
¼ cup bread crumbs,
  toasted

Preheat oven to 375°F. Sift flour, baking powder, and salt into small bowl. With electric beater, cut in 3 tablespoons margarine on lowest speed; then turn to medium speed for about 5 minutes until mixture is well blended and resembles small peas. Add ½ cup nonfat milk mixed with coloring and ½ cup sweetener. Continue beating on medium speed for about 1 minute; batter will be stiff. Add remaining nonfat milk; beat for a minute, then add unbeaten egg and beat one more minute. Pour into greased 8″ round cake pan. Mix remaining tablespoon margarine, cinnamon, and toasted bread crumbs and sprinkle on top of dough. Bake until cake springs back when lightly touched (about 20 minutes).

PAULA'S POPOVERS

Exchanges per serving: 1 popover = 1½ Starch, 1 Fat,
                                   ½ Medium-Fat Meat
Calories per serving: 218   Yield: 8 popovers

2 cups flour
1 teaspoon salt
4 eggs

2 cups nonfat milk
6 tablespoons diet
  margarine, melted

Preheat oven to 350°F. Sift flour and salt. Beat eggs slightly; add milk and margarine; beat until blended. Gradually add dry ingredients. Grease ramekin cups well; fill about ¾ full. Bake 1 hour and 10 minutes; remove from oven. Slit each side quickly to release steam. Return to oven until brown and crisp and tops are firm. Lift out of ramekins; serve hot.

COFFEE CAKE, CHOCOLATE STYLE

Exchanges per serving: one ½″ slice = 1 Starch, 1 Fat (if using sour half-and-half, add ½ Fat),
¼ Medium-Fat Meat

Calories per serving: 170 (155 if using plain yogurt) Yield: 12 servings

⅔ cup diet margarine
Nonnutritive sweetener equivalent to 1 cup sugar
3 eggs
1 teaspoon orange peel, grated
1 cup imitation sour cream, sour half-and-half, or plain yogurt
1 teaspoon vanilla extract
¼ teaspoon salt
½ teaspoon baking soda

1½ teaspoons baking powder
2 cups + 2 teaspoons flour
1 ounce unsweetened chocolate
Nonnutritive sweetener equivalent to ½ cup brown sugar
1 teaspoon cinnamon
1 tablespoon diet margarine

Preheat oven to 350°F. Cream margarine and sweetener until light and fluffy; add eggs one at a time, beating each until smooth. Mix in orange peel, sour cream, and vanilla. Stir salt, baking soda, baking powder, and 2 cups flour together; blend with creamed mixture thoroughly. Place in a well-greased 10″ tube pan. Melt chocolate over double boiler and swirl over batter with spoon to form ripples through batter. Mix brown sugar substitute, cinnamon, and softened margarine with remaining 2 tablespoons flour; sprinkle over batter. Bake until tester inserted in center comes out clean (50–60 minutes).

STUFFING
(For chicken, turkey, or meat)

Exchanges per serving: 1 cup = 1 Starch, ⅔ Fat
Calories per serving: 125   Yield: 6 servings

½ cup celery, chopped fine   ¼ cup diet margarine
½ cup onion, chopped fine   8-ounce package herb-
½ cup mushrooms,   seasoned stuffing mix
  chopped fine   1 cup boiling water

Sauté celery, onion, and mushrooms in margarine until onion is
golden. Add stuffing mix to boiling water, then toss all together.
Mix well.

SEEDED STUFFING
(For chicken, turkey, or meat)

Exchanges per serving: ½ cup = 1 Starch, ½ Fat, ⅔ Vegetable
Calories per serving: 85   Yield: 6 cups

1 onion, chopped fine   8-ounce package stuffing
2 stalks celery, chopped   mix
  fine   ¼ teaspoon each: celery,
1 cup mushrooms,   sesame, and poppy seeds
  chopped fine   1 cup boiling water
2 tablespoons diet
  margarine

Sauté onion, celery, and mushrooms in margarine until onion is
golden. Add stuffing mix and seeds to boiling water; mix all ingredients together.

MARVELOUS MARMALADE STUFFING

Exchanges per serving: ½ cup = 2 Starch, 2½ Fat

Calories per serving: 261   Yield: 3 cups

8-ounce package
  cornbread stuffing
½ cup diet margarine,
  melted
½ cup celery, chopped fine

¼ cup onion, chopped fine
¼ cup almonds, slivered
  and chopped
½ cup dietetic marmalade

Mix all ingredients; toss lightly but thoroughly. Use to lightly stuff a 4- to 5-pound chicken.

DESSERTS:
FRUITS, PUDDINGS,
AND SOUFFLÉS

NOTE
Desserts really should be used infrequently—as opposed to never!

LUCY'S LUSCIOUS APRICOT
SOUFFLÉ DESSERT

Exchanges per serving: 1 serving = ½ Fruit, 1 Lean Meat
Calories per serving: 73   Yield: 8 servings

1 cup dried apricots	2 cups egg whites (10–12)
Nonnutritive sweetener	Dash of salt
equivalent to 1¼ cups	1 cup low-calorie nondairy
sugar	whipped topping
Water to cover	

Preheat oven to 300°F. Combine apricots and ¾ cup sweetener in a saucepan; add sufficient water to cover. Cook slowly until sweetener dissolves, stirring occasionally; cover pan and cook over low heat until apricots are tender and plump; drain. Retain syrup. Puree apricots. Beat egg whites, which should be at room temperature, with salt until egg whites are stiff; add remaining ½ cup sweetener. Fold in pureed apricots, mixing thoroughly. Turn into buttered tube pan. Bake 45 minutes. The soufflé will rise and become golden brown. Top with nondairy whip, to which 2 tablespoons apricot syrup have been added after whipping.

BAKED FRESH PEACHES

Exchanges per serving: 1 peach = 1 Fruit
Calories per serving: 60   Yield: 4 servings

4 peaches
1 teaspoon diet margarine

Nonnutritive sweetener
equivalent to ½ cup
sugar
1 tablespoon lemon juice

Preheat oven to 350°F. Cut about an inch of skin from each end of peach; set in a baking dish that has been well greased with margarine. Sprinkle with sweetener and lemon juice. Bake about 20 minutes; serve cold or hot, with milk or cream if desired.

2 tablespoons light cream = 45 calories
4 tablespoons nonfat milk = 23 calories

BANANA FREEZE

Exchanges per serving: 1 cup = 1 Fruit
Calories per serving: 63   Yield: 6 cups

3 bananas, crushed
Nonnutritive sweetener
equivalent to 2
tablespoons sugar

1 cup unsweetened orange
juice
1 teaspoon lemon juice
¼ cup water

Combine all ingredients, mixing well. Divide mixture evenly into 6 paper cups and freeze until firm. Let stand at room temperature 5–6 minutes; peel paper cup as freeze is being eaten.

DIETETIC SPICED PEACHES

Exchanges per serving: 1 serving = 1 Fruit
Calories per serving: 60   Yield: 2 servings

    4 dietetic peach halves   1 cup liquid from peaches
    16 whole cloves

Preheat oven to 375°F. Place peaches in small baking pan, pitted
side up. Stick 4 cloves in each half; pour liquid over fruit. Bake
20 minutes. Serve hot.

SUMMER FRUIT MIX

Exchanges per serving: ¾ cup = 1 Fruit
Calories per serving: 60   Yield: 5 cups

    2 cups strawberries   Nonnutritive sweetener
    1 cup grapes   equivalent to ¼ cup
    1 cup melon balls   sugar
    1 cup blackberries

Wash and clean fruit; combine with sweetener; chill. This goes
well topped with Custard Sauce for Shortcakes (see Index).

APPLESAUCE, UNCOOKED

Exchanges per serving: 1 cup = 1 Fruit
Calories per serving: 60   Yield: 4 cups

    2 cups apples, washed,   Dash of cloves
      cored, and cubed, but not   Dash of ginger
      peeled   ¼ teaspoon nutmeg
    2 cups cold water   2 drops red vegetable food
    3 tablespoons lemon juice   coloring (optional)
    Nonnutritive sweetener
      equivalent to 3 teaspoons
      sugar

As you cut apples, place them in bowl with water and lemon
juice. Remove ½ cup juice from bowl; to it add sweetener,

spices, and half the apple cubes. Blend; then add the additional cubes gradually until all is smoothly blended. Add coloring.

SPICED FRUIT

Exchanges per serving: 1 cup = 2 Fruit
Calories per serving: 88   Yield: 5 cups

1 cup dietetic pineapple juice	2 cups dietetic pear halves
¼ teaspoon cinnamon	2 cups dietetic peach halves

Heat pineapple juice and cinnamon to boil; chill fruit, from which syrup has been drained; place in a bowl. Pour pineapple juice over fruit; serve at once.

WINE SAUCE WITH FRUIT

Exchanges per serving: 1 serving = ½ Fat, 2 Fruit
Calories per serving: 149   Yield: 4 servings

4 cups apples, peeled and sliced (or substitute other fruit, such as bananas, peaches, pears)	1 cup red wine
	½ tablespoon arrowroot
	Nonnutritive sweetener equivalent to 1 cup sugar
2 tablespoons diet margarine	Dash of allspice

Brown apples in margarine. Add wine to arrowroot a little at a time to make a smooth paste. Add sweetener; cook over medium heat, stirring constantly, until clear and thick; add allspice. Pour over fruit slices and simmer a few minutes. Serve immediately.

HAWAIIAN FRUIT FRITTERS

Exchanges per serving: 1 fritter = ¼ Starch, ¼ Fruit
Calories per serving: 45   Yield: 20 fritters

2 eggs
½ cup nonfat milk
½ teaspoon seasoned salt

2 cups fresh pineapple (or
  papaya or banana)
  (approximately ten 1″
  pieces per cup)
2 cups cornflakes, finely
  crushed

Preheat oven to 425°F. Beat eggs, nonfat milk, and salt together; cut fruit into inch-long pieces and dip in egg mixture; roll in cornflakes. Put on cookie sheet; bake for 5–10 minutes, until golden. Serve with Hot Shoyu (Soy) Sauce dip (see Index).

POLLY'S PEAR DISH

Exchanges per serving: 1 slice = 1 Starch, 1 Fat, 2 Fruit
Calories per serving: 205   Yield: 8 servings

½ cup water
Nonnutritive sweetener
  equivalent to 1 cup sugar
1 tablespoon fresh lemon
  juice
8 fresh pears, pared, cored,
  and sliced thin

8″ pie shell, unbaked
1 cup low-calorie apricot
  preserves
Dash of nutmeg
Dash of allspice

Preheat oven to 425°F. Combine water, sweetener, and lemon juice in saucepan. Add pear slices a few at a time; cook gently until tender (about 5–6 minutes). Cool a little, then drain, saving ¼ cup liquid. Place pear slices in circle in unbaked pie shell. Bake until golden brown; cool. Combine apricot preserves and reserved liquid in a saucepan; heat until bubbly, then force through sieve. Spoon over pear slices to glaze; sprinkle with nutmeg and allspice. Chill.

BAKED APPLES

Exchanges per serving: 1 apple = 1 Fruit
Calories per serving: 60   Yield: 2 servings

2 medium apples   Dash of cinnamon
  (approximately 5 ounces   Dash of allspice
  each)   4 tablespoons dietetic
2 teaspoons lemon juice   maple topping
Dash of nutmeg

Preheat oven to 350°F. Core apples and peel about ½ of each apple; sprinkle lemon juice over cut surfaces. Dust apple with mixture of nutmeg, cinnamon, and allspice. Fill cavity with dietetic maple topping; bake covered about 25 minutes. Remove cover and continue baking until apples are tender.

MARTI'S APPLE CRISP

Exchanges per serving: 1 serving = ½ Fat, 1 Fruit, ½ Starch,
                                     ⅔ Lean Meat
Calories per serving: 150   Yield: 6 servings

4 apples, cored, peeled,   ½ cup flour
  and sliced   ½ teaspoon cinnamon
¼ cup water   ½ teaspoon allspice
½ teaspoon fresh lemon   ½ teaspoon salt
  juice   3 tablespoons diet
Nonnutritive sweetener   margarine
  equivalent to ⅔ cup   ½ cup Parmesan cheese,
  sugar   grated

Preheat oven to 325°F. Grease a shallow baking dish; place apple slices on bottom. Combine water, lemon juice, and sweetener; pour over apples. Combine dry ingredients; cut in margarine until mixture is the consistency of large peas; sprinkle over apples. If desired, cover with grated cheese.

DIETETIC APPLE CRUNCH

Exchanges per serving: 1 serving = ⅓ Starch, ½ Fruit
Calories per serving: 65   Yield: 6 servings

2 slices dry bread	3 cups apples, cored and
1 tablespoon diet	sliced
margarine	1 tablespoon lemon juice
½ teaspoon cinnamon	¾ cup dietetic maple syrup
½ teaspoon allspice	

Preheat oven to 350°F. Make crumbs from bread and toast in oven. Mix toasted crumbs with margarine, cinnamon, and ¼ teaspoon allspice. Mix apples with lemon juice, maple syrup, and remainder of allspice; spread in well-greased shallow baking dish (approximately 8″ round). Cover with crumb mixture; bake 45 minutes, or until apple slices are tender. Serve warm.

TASTY APPLESAUCE

Exchanges per serving: 1 serving = ¼ Fruit,
                                  ½ Medium-Fat Meat
Calories per serving: 50   Yield: 4 servings

4 teaspoons cinnamon	½ cup unsweetened
1 teaspoon salt	applesauce
1 teaspoon vanilla	2 egg whites
Nonnutritive sweetener	Dash of allspice
equivalent to ¼ cup	
sugar	

Stir first five ingredients together. Place in refrigerator until chilled. Before serving, beat egg whites to form stiff peaks; fold applesauce mix into whites and sprinkle with allspice.

FRUIT CAKE PUDDING

Exchanges per serving: 1 serving = ¼ Starch, ½ Medium-Fat
                                                  Meat, ¼ Nonfat Milk
Calories per serving: 85   Yield: 6 servings

3 eggs, separated	Nonnutritive sweetener
1 tablespoon fresh citrus fruit peel, grated	equivalent to 6 tablespoons sugar
¼ cup fresh citrus fruit juice	¼ cup flour, sifted
1⅓ cups nonfat milk	Dash of salt

Preheat oven to 325°F. Beat egg whites until stiff peaks form;
set aside. Add fruit peel and juice to yolks, beating at medium
speed until well blended. Add nonfat milk; beat about 1 minute
at low speed. Add remaining ingredients; beat again at low
speed until smooth. Fold into egg whites. Spoon into custard
cups; place cups in baking pan filled with about 1″ water. Bake
until lightly browned on top (about 45 minutes). Serve hot or
cold.

FRUIT MOUNTAIN

Exchanges per serving: 1 serving = ½ Starch, ¾ Fruit,
                                                  ⅓ Skim Milk
Calories per serving: 115   Yield: 6 servings

1 envelope low-calorie vanilla pudding and pie filling mix	8-ounce dietetic cherry or apple pie filling (Sego or other dietetic pie filling)
2 cups nonfat milk	Cinnamon
1 teaspoon almond extract	

Prepare pudding according to directions on package, using
nonfat milk; add almond extract. Divide into 6 dessert glasses;
cool. Top with pie filling and sprinkle with cinnamon.

LEMON PUDDING

Exchanges per serving: 1 cup = 2 Fat, 2 Medium-Fat Meat
Calories per serving: 240   Yield: 4 servings

Nonnutritive sweetener
equivalent to 1½ cups
sugar
½ cup diet margarine

2 tablespoons lemon peel
8 eggs
1 cup lemon juice

Combine all ingredients in top of double boiler; cook over boiling water until thick, stirring constantly. Cover and store in refrigerator until cool.

OLGA'S FRUIT FESTIVAL

Exchanges per serving: 1 serving = ½ Fat, 1 Fruit
Calories per serving: 102   Yield: 8 servings

2 cups strawberries,
washed and hulled
3 cups fresh peaches,
peeled and sliced
2 cups seedless green
grapes

Nonnutritive sweetener
equivalent to ⅔ cup
sugar
¼ cup orange curaçao
½ cup nondairy whipped
topping
1 ounce unsweetened
chocolate, well grated

Sprinkle strawberries over peaches; add grapes, sweetener, and curaçao. Refrigerate overnight. Prior to serving, heat broiler. Place fruit in heatproof dessert dishes; top with whipped topping. Sprinkle top with grated chocolate; place under broiler about 30 seconds, or just until chocolate melts. Serve at once.

FRUIT WHIP

Exchanges per serving: 1 cup = ½ Skim Milk
Calories per serving: 45   Yield: 6 servings

1½ tablespoons unflavored   Nonnutritive sweetener
  gelatin   equivalent to ¼ cup
3 cups nonfat milk   sugar
                       2 teaspoons any fruit
                       extract

Sprinkle gelatin over nonfat milk in saucepan; cook over low
heat until gelatin dissolves. Add sweetener and fruit extract.
Chill in refrigerator until mixture is consistency of egg white.
Remove from refrigerator and beat at highest speed of mixer
until mixture is doubled in volume (this will be very fluffy).
Place in a mold and refrigerate until set. May be garnished with
slice of favorite fruit, if desired.

APRICOT OR PRUNE FRUIT SNOW

Exchanges per serving: 1 serving = ½ Fruit
Calories per serving: 40   Yield: 6 servings

1 envelope lemon-flavored   1 egg white
  low-calorie gelatin   6 pieces unsweetened
1 cup boiling water   dried apricots or prunes
1 cup unsweetened apple   3 teaspoons almonds,
  juice or apricot nectar   slivered

Dissolve gelatin in boiling water. Add juice; cool. Chill until
syrupy. Add egg white and beat until frothy. Fill 6 dessert
glasses with "snow." Chill until firm; decorate each with apricot
or prune and sprinkle ½ teaspoon slivered almonds over fruit.

FRUIT COCKTAIL CAKE DESSERT

Exchanges per serving: 1 section = ½ Starch, ¾ Fruit,
                                                      ½ Lean Meat

Calories per serving: 112   Yield: 10 sections

Nonnutritive sweetener
  equivalent to ½ cup
  sugar
1 tablespoon unflavored
  gelatin
¼ teaspoon salt
½ cup water
4 cups dietetic fruit
  cocktail

1 tablespoon lemon juice
4–5 drops almond extract
2 eggs whites
1 cup nondairy whipped
  topping
10 ladyfingers, split (these
  can be made from Aunt
  Jeanne's Sponge Cake*)

Combine sweetener, gelatin, and salt; add ½ cup water and cook, stirring, over medium heat until gelatin dissolves. Chill until partially set. Drain fruit cocktail; add lemon juice and almond extract. Put gelatin mixture, egg whites, and half the fruit cocktail in a large mixing bowl. Start mixer on low speed, then turn to high and beat 10 minutes, until fluffy; chill until partially set. Fold in remaining fruit cocktail and whipped topping. Line sides of springform pan with ladyfingers. Pour filling in carefully; chill overnight. Remove sides of pan to serve.

* 10 pieces of finger-shaped slices of Aunt Jeanne's Sponge Cake, each cut into quarters. See Index.

FRUIT CRISP

Exchanges per serving: 1 serving = ½ Starch, ⅓ Fat, 1 Fruit
Calories per serving: 101   Yield: 6 servings

4 cups fruit, peeled and
   sliced thin (apples,
   peaches, apricots)
Nonnutritive sweetener
   equivalent to ⅔ cup
   sugar
1 teaspoon fresh lemon
   juice

½ cup quick-cooking
   rolled oats
Nonnutritive sweetener
   equivalent to 2
   tablespoons brown sugar
2 tablespoons arrowroot
¼ teaspoon allspice
2 tablespoons diet
   margarine

Preheat oven to 350°F. Combine fruit with half of a sweetener
(equivalent to ⅓ cup white sugar) and juice. Place in casserole.
Combine oats, brown sugar substitute, arrowroot, allspice, and
remainder of regular sugar substitute. Cut in margarine until
crumbly; sprinkle evenly over fruit. Bake about 1 hour, or until
tender. Serve hot or cold.

MOCHA SURPRISE

Exchanges per serving: 1 cup = None
Calories per serving: 28   Yield: 3 cups

2 envelopes unflavored
   gelatin
½ cup cold water
3 cups very strong coffee
Nonnutritive sweetener
   equivalent to ⅓ cup
   sugar

½ teaspoon vanilla
Dash of salt
3 tablespoons nondairy
   whipped topping

Soften gelatin in water in a medium-size pan. Heat, stirring
constantly, until dissolved. Stir in coffee, sweetener, vanilla, and
salt. Pour into an 8″ square pan; chill 2 hours. Put gelatin
through potato ricer (or sieve) and spoon into 3 dessert dishes.
Decorate each with 1 tablespoon nondairy whipped topping.

CHOCOLATE BISQUE CAPRI

Exchanges per serving: 2-ounce scoop = 1 Fat
Calories per serving: 45 + ice cream   Yield: 16 servings

½ cup toasted almonds,   ½ teaspoon almond extract
   chopped   1 quart dietetic chocolate
⅓ cup toasted coconut,   ice cream, softened
   chopped

Combine almonds and coconut; reserving 2 tablespoons for topping, fold remainder and almond extract quickly into ice cream. Place in small paper dessert cups and sprinkle with topping. Keep in freezer until ready to serve.

FRUIT SOUFFLÉ

Exchanges per serving: ½ cup = ¾ Fruit
Calories per serving: 45   Yield: 6 servings

1 envelope unflavored   2 cups unsweetened,
   gelatin   pureed fruit (apples,
1 cup cold water   pears, pineapple), canned
1 teaspoon lemon rind,   or cooked
   finely grated

Sprinkle gelatin on ½ cup water; soften a few minutes. Stir over low heat about 3 minutes until gelatin is dissolved; add remaining water, rind, and fruit. Chill until thick enough to mound on spoon. Beat until very light; pour into a soufflé dish and chill until firm.

LOW-CALORIE COFFEE CREAM MOUSSE

Exchanges per serving: 1 serving = ¼ Fat, ¼ Medium-Fat Meat
Calories per serving: 61   Yield: 12 servings

2 envelopes unflavored
  gelatin
2 cups cold coffee, double
  strength
3 eggs, separated
Nonnutritive sweetener
  equivalent to ¾ cup
  sugar

1 ounce semisweet
  chocolate chips
3 tablespoons rum or
  brandy flavoring
2 cups nondairy whipped
  topping

Sprinkle gelatin over 1 cup coffee in small bowl; let soften about
5 minutes. Using a rotary beater, beat egg yolks with sweetener
equivalent to ½ cup sugar until light, in the top of a double
boiler. Once light, beat in remaining coffee, chocolate chips, and
softened gelatin. Stir constantly over simmering water until
chocolate is melted and coats a metal spoon (about 10 minutes).
Remove from heat; stir in flavoring. Set top of double boiler in
ice and cool, stirring often, until mixture becomes as thick as
unbeaten egg white. Beat egg whites until soft peaks form when
beaters are raised; gradually beat in remaining sweetener, until
whites are stiff and glossy. Fold gelatin mixture into 1 cup prepared whipped topping; fold in whites gently, until well
blended. Place in large mold that has been rinsed well in cold
water. Place in refrigerator until firm (5–6 hours). To unmold,
run knife around edge of mold; invert over serving platter.
Place hot, damp cloth over mold and shake gently to release; lift
off mold. Spoon 1 cup nondairy whipped topping on dessert
mold before serving.

PEAR PUDDING DORIS

Exchanges per serving: 3 slices = ⅓ Medium-Fat Meat, ½ Fruit
Calories per serving: 80   Yield: 6 servings

6 tablespoons nonfat dry milk

1 cup water

1 envelope unflavored gelatin

5-ounce jar low-calorie chocolate topping

2 egg whites

1 jar unsweetened pear slices

Dissolve dry milk in ¾ cup water; on remaining ¼ cup water sprinkle gelatin to soften. Mix milk with gelatin; stir over low heat until gelatin dissolves; add chocolate topping. Cool until mixture thickens enough to mound on a spoon. Beat egg whites stiff; fold in drained pears well and line dessert dishes with 3 slices in each dish. Add chocolate mixture and chill until firm.

CAKES

LORENE'S CHEESECAKE

Exchanges per serving: 1 wedge = ¾ Fat, ⅓ Very Lean Meat,
⅔ Lean Meat

Calories per serving: 115   Yield: 24 wedges

¾ cup diet margarine
Nonnutritive sweetener
  equivalent to 1¼ cups
  sugar
4 eggs
2 cups low-fat cottage
  cheese
3 tablespoons arrowroot

2 cups Neufchâtel cheese
  (2 8-ounce packages)
6 level tablespoons flour
1 cup imitation sour cream
  or sour half-and-half
½ teaspoon vanilla extract
½ teaspoon lemon juice
1 cup artificially sweetened
  crushed pineapple

Preheat oven to 350°F. Cream first two ingredients; add eggs, cottage cheese, arrowroot, and Neufchâtel; blend well after each addition. Add flour, sour cream, vanilla, lemon juice, and crushed pineapple, stirring well. Pour into springform pan. Bake 2 hours. When baking, dough will rise over edge but will not run out. Leave in oven for 2 hours with heat off; keep in refrigerator overnight.

SPICE AND MAPLE CAKE

Exchanges per serving: 1½″ slice = ½ Starch,
                                ½ Medium-Fat Meat

Calories per serving: 88   Yield: 10 servings

1 cup flour	2 eggs, separated
¼ cup nonfat dry milk	3 egg yolks
1 teaspoon baking powder	½ cup maple-flavored
1 teaspoon cinnamon	topping*
1 teaspoon nutmeg	½ teaspoon cream of tartar
¼ teaspoon salt	

Preheat oven to 325°F. Sift first six ingredients together three times. Mix five egg yolks, slightly beaten, with maple topping; beat at top speed of mixer until light and fluffy (about 10 minutes). Beat two egg whites slightly; add cream of tartar; continue to beat until whites hold a stiff peak. Fold sifted dry ingredients carefully, a small amount at a time, into egg yolk mixture. Gently fold in egg whites; pour into 9″ tube pan at once. Bake about 35 minutes, or until cake springs back when lightly touched. Invert pan and let hang until cool.

DELIGHTFUL CHEESECAKE

Exchanges per serving: 1 serving = 1 Lean Meat
Calories per serving: 85   Yield: 9 servings

4 tablespoons graham cracker crumbs	1½ cups low-fat cottage cheese
2 envelopes unflavored gelatin	3 eggs, separated
Water	¼ cup nonfat milk
1 cup low-calorie pineapple tidbits, reserving juice	2 tablespoons lemon juice
	Nonnutritive sweetener equivalent to ½ cup sugar
	1 teaspoon vanilla extract
	¼ teaspoon salt

* Use Low-Calorie Whipped Topping and add 4 or 5 drops of maple flavoring.

Sprinkle 3 tablespoons graham cracker crumbs on bottom of 9″ pie or cake pan; set aside. Soften gelatin in ½ cup water. Add water to pineapple juice to make ¾ cup; bring to a boil; stir in gelatin. In bowl, beat cottage cheese until nearly smooth, at highest speed on mixer (about 3–4 minutes). Add egg yolks, nonfat milk, lemon juice, sweetener, vanilla, and salt; beat well. Blend in gelatin at low speed. Chill. Stir occasionally until mixture is thick, but not set (about 1 hour). Beat whites at highest speed until soft peaks form; fold in gelatin mixture by hand. Spoon over crumbs in pan; sprinkle remaining tablespoon of crumbs over filling. Add pineapple tidbits on top; chill overnight in refrigerator.

NO-CRUST CHEESECAKE

Exchanges per serving: 1 wedge = ¾ Fat, 1 Lean Meat
Calories per serving: 100   Yield: 24 wedges

2 cups low-fat cottage cheese

2 cups Neufchâtel cheese, creamed

Nonnutritive sweetener equivalent to 1½ cups sugar

3 eggs

1½ tablespoons lemon juice

1 teaspoon vanilla extract

½ cup diet margarine, melted

1½ tablespoons arrowroot

3 tablespoons flour

2 cups imitation sour cream or sour half-and-half

Preheat oven to 325°F. Cream the cheeses together, gradually adding sweetener, beating after each addition. Add eggs, beat well; add lemon juice, vanilla, and margarine. Mix arrowroot and flour with enough sour cream to make a smooth paste. Add paste and remaining sour cream to cheese mixture; blend thoroughly. Pour into greased 9″ springform pan. Bake 1 hour or longer, until firm; turn off oven. Let cake remain in oven 2 hours or longer. Place in refrigerator overnight. Serve cold.

BANANA RAISIN CAKE

Exchanges per serving: 1 slice = ½ Starch, ½ Fat, ½ Fruit
Calories per serving: 118   Yield: 18 slices

2 cups flour
1½ teaspoons baking powder
Nonnutritive sweetener equivalent to 1½ cups sugar
1 teaspoon baking soda
1 teaspoon salt
½ cup diet margarine
1 cup bananas (about 3), mashed
¼ cup nonfat milk
1 teaspoon lemon peel, grated
1 teaspoon vanilla extract
2 eggs
1 cup white raisins, chopped
½ cup nuts, chopped fine

Preheat oven to 350°F. Sift flour, baking powder, sweetener, baking soda, and salt. Add margarine, bananas, nonfat milk, lemon peel, and vanilla; beat 3 minutes on electric mixer at medium speed, scraping bowl constantly. Add eggs; beat 2 minutes more, continuing to scrape bowl frequently. Stir in raisins and nuts. Pour batter into a well-greased and lightly floured 12″ × 9″ × 2″ pan. Bake until cake tests done. Turn out on rack to cool after 5 minutes.

CHOCOLATE CAKE

Exchanges per serving: 1 serving = ½ Starch, ⅓ Fat
Calories per serving: 66 (frosting not included) Yield: 8 servings

¾ cup flour, sifted
¼ teaspoon salt
1 teaspoon baking powder
¼ teaspoon baking soda
3 tablespoons unsweetened cocoa
¼ cup cold coffee
1 egg
Nonnutritive sweetener equivalent to ½ cup sugar
¼ cup water
1 tablespoon salad oil
1 teaspoon vanilla extract

Preheat oven to 350°F. Line an 8″ round layer cake pan with paper; grease lightly with margarine. Sift first four ingredients together; blend in cocoa and coffee. Beat egg, sweetener, water, oil, and vanilla. Stir into first mixture; mix until smooth. Pour batter into pan, cover with foil, and place in shallow pan of water. Bake about 30 minutes. Remove from pan; cool on cake rack. Cut crosswise, fill, and frost with desired frosting.

CHARLOTTE'S CHOCOLATE CAKE

Exchanges per serving: 1 serving = ¾ Starch, ½ Fat

Calories per serving: 100   Yield: 9 servings

⅓ cup diet margarine, softened

Nonnutritive sweetener equivalent to ¼ cup brown sugar

1 egg

Nonnutritive sweetener equivalent to ⅓ cup sugar

1⅓ cups flour

3 tablespoons unsweetened cocoa

2 teaspoons baking powder

½ teaspoon baking soda

½ cup nonfat milk

½ teaspoon vanilla extract

½ teaspoon almond extract

2 tablespoons nuts, chopped fine

Preheat oven to 350°F. Mix margarine, brown sugar substitute, egg, and regular sugar substitute; beat at high speed two minutes, scraping bowl occasionally. Add flour, cocoa, baking powder, baking soda, nonfat milk, and extracts; blend at low speed about 2 minutes (batter will be thick). Spread batter in a well-greased 8″ layer pan; sprinkle with nuts. Bake until tester inserted in center comes out clean.

CHOCOLATE CHIFFON CAKE WITH RUM

Exchanges per serving: 1 slice = 1 Starch, 2 Fat,
                                ½ Medium-Fat Meat

Calories per serving: 200   Yield: 12 slices

8 eggs	1½ teaspoons baking soda
½ cup cocoa	1¾ cups flour
¾ cup boiling water	½ cup soy oil
Nonnutritive sweetener	2 tablespoons rum extract
equivalent to 1¾ cups	½ teaspoon cream of tartar
sugar	

Preheat oven to 325°F. Let eggs reach room temperature, then separate. Combine cocoa and water in small bowl. Stir until smooth; cool. Sift sweetener, baking soda, and flour into large bowl; make well in center; add oil, egg yolks, rum extract, and cocoa mixture; beat until smooth. Add cream of tartar to egg whites; beat very stiff. Pour batter over whites; gently fold until just blended. Bake in ungreased Bundt pan (or 10″ tube pan) until straw inserted comes out clean. Cool cake completely; remove from pan. Serve plain or with nondairy whipped topping (calories and exchanges not included for topping).

LOU'S LIGHT CAKE

Exchanges per serving: 1 serving = 1½ Fat, 2 Starch
Calories per serving: 229   Yield: 10 servings

⅔ cup diet margarine	1½ cups cold water
Nonnutritive sweetener	3½ cups flour, sifted
equivalent to 2 cups	½ teaspoon salt
sugar	4 teaspoons baking
2 teaspoons vanilla extract	powder
2 teaspoons boiling water	¾ cup (4–5) egg whites

Preheat oven to 350°F. Cream margarine and sweetener; add vanilla and boiling water; blend thoroughly. Add cold water; beat 1 minute. Sift flour and salt four times; add bit by bit, alternating with small amounts of water mixture, beating well after each addition. Beat egg whites until stiff. Sift baking powder over top of batter and fold in gently with egg whites. Bake in two well-greased and floured 10″ pans until done, or when tester comes out clean.

PAM'S QUICK LAYER CAKE

Exchanges per serving: 1 wedge = 1 Starch, 2 Fat
Calories per serving: 198   Yield: 12 wedges

Nonnutritive sweetener
  equivalent to 1 cup sugar
Dash of salt
2 cups flour
3 teaspoons baking
  powder
⅓ cup diet margarine

1 egg
¾ cup nonfat milk
½ teaspoon vanilla extract
½ teaspoon almond extract
1 cup pecans, chopped
  extra fine

Preheat oven to 375°F. Sift sweetener, salt, flour, and baking powder together three or four times. Cut in margarine with pastry blender or knife until mixture resembles cornmeal. Beat egg until lemon-colored and thick; add nonfat milk and extracts. Add to first mixture gradually. Add nuts and stir well. Pour into two well-greased 8″ layer pans. Bake about 25 minutes or until tester comes out clean. Cool; remove cake from pans. Cool further on wire rack.

SOUTHERN HOSPITALITY CAKE

Exchanges per serving: 1 wedge = 1 Starch, ½ Fat, ½ Fruit
Calories per serving: 117   Yield: 9 wedges

⅓ cup diet margarine, softened	1 teaspoon baking powder
	½ teaspoon baking soda
Nonnutritive sweetener equivalent to ¾ cup sugar	½ teaspoon orange extract
	⅔ cup fresh orange juice
	⅓ cup raisins
1 egg	2 tablespoons nuts, chopped fine
1⅓ cups flour	

Preheat oven to 350°F. Combine margarine, sweetener, and egg; beat 2 minutes on high speed of mixer. Scrape bowl occasionally. Add flour, baking powder, baking soda, orange extract, and juice; blend at low speed about 2 minutes (batter will be fairly thick). Stir in raisins; spread batter in a well-greased 8″ layer pan. Sprinkle nuts on top. Bake until golden brown (about 30 minutes or until tester comes out clean).

FAMILY FAVORITE CAKE

Exchanges per serving: 1 wedge = 1 Starch, ¾ Fat
Calories per serving: 146   Yield: 15 wedges

¾ cup diet margarine	½ teaspoon salt
Nonnutritive sweetener equivalent to 1½ cups sugar	3 cups flour
	1 cup nonfat milk
	1 teaspoon almond extract
4 teaspoons baking powder	¾ cup egg whites

Preheat oven to 375°F. Cream margarine and sweetener. Sift baking powder, salt, and flour. Add alternately with nonfat milk to creamed mixture; add almond extract. Beat egg whites until stiff peaks form; fold in. Pour into two well-greased 9″ layer pans. Bake about 30 minutes. Cool a few minutes; remove from pans; cool further on wire rack.

ORANGE CHIFFON CAKE

Exchanges per serving: 1½″ slice = 1 Starch, 1½ Fat,
⅓ Medium-Fat Meat

Calories per serving: 168   Yield: 16 squares

8 egg whites
5 egg yolks
½ teaspoon cream of tartar
2¼ cups flour, sifted
3 teaspoons baking powder
1 teaspoon salt
Nonnutritive sweetener equivalent to 1½ cups sugar

½ cup salad oil
3 tablespoons orange peel, finely grated
Artificial sweetener equivalent to ¼ cup sugar added to ¾ cup orange juice

Preheat over to 325°F. Bring eggs to room temperature. Add cream of tartar to egg whites; beat until they stand in peaks (stiffer than for meringue). Sift dry ingredients; make a well in center; add salad oil, egg yolks, peel, and juice-sweetener mixture; stir to blend. Beat one minute at medium speed. Add yolk-orange mixture to whites slowly, folding these together until smooth and completely mixed. Pour into an 8″ square cake pan that has been rinsed (shake out excess water). Bake until cake is pale golden brown and a cake tester comes out clean (about 30 minutes or a little more). Invert pan and cool. When cake pan is cool enough to handle (but not cold), run a knife around edges of pan; then, with fingertips, carefully pull cake away from edges, lifting slightly to loosen bottom. Cool on rack. Cut into serving pieces.

ORANGE CAKE

Exchanges per serving: 1 slice = ½ Starch, 1 Fat, ½ Medium-
Fat Meat, ⅓ Fruit

Calories per serving: 142   Yield: 10 slices

1 cup flour
1½ teaspoons baking
powder
½ teaspoon salt
¼ cup oil
4 eggs, separated

½ cup unsweetened frozen
orange juice concentrate
Nonnutritive sweetener
equivalent to 1½ cups
sugar
¼ teaspoon cr   of tartar

Preheat oven to 350°F. Sift flour, baking powder, and salt together. Set aside one egg yolk.* Add, in order, oil, 3 egg yolks,
orange juice concentrate, and sweetener; beat until smooth.
Add cream of tartar to egg whites and beat until stiff. Add egg
yolk mixture to whites; fold in gently until blended, but do not
overmix. Pour into 9″ tube pan; bake 35 minutes.

LOU'S CHIFFON CAKE

Exchanges per serving: 1 serving = 1 Starch, 2 Fat,
⅓ Medium-Fat Meat

Calories per serving: 200   Yield: 12 servings

1 teaspoon salt
2¼ cups flour, sifted
3 teaspoons baking
powder
½ cup salad oil
4 eggs, separated
½ cup water

Nonnutritive sweetener
equivalent to 1½ cups
sugar
2 teaspoons lemon rind,
grated
1 teaspoon vanilla extract
½ teaspoon cream of tartar

Preheat oven to 325°F. Sift salt, flour, and baking powder. Add
oil, well-beaten egg yolks, water, sweetener, rind, and vanilla.
Beat until smooth. Beat egg whites until stiff; add cream of tartar; beat until very stiff peaks form. Gently fold batter into egg

* Refrigerate for future use.

whites until just blended (do not stir). Place in ungreased 9″ tube pan. Bake until done (about 1 hour). Invert cake to cool.

MARGARET'S POUND CAKE

Exchanges per serving: 1½″ slice = 1½ Starch, 2 Fat,
½ Medium-Fat Meat

Calories per serving: 248   Yield: 15 servings

1 teaspoon salt
4 cups flour
½ teaspoon cream of tartar
2 cups diet margarine

Nonnutritive sweetener
equivalent to 2 cups
sugar
8 eggs
1 teaspoon vanilla extract
½ teaspoon allspice

Preheat oven to 325°F. Sift salt, flour, and cream of tartar; set aside. Cream margarine until fluffy; add sweetener gradually; continue to cream until very fluffy. Beat in eggs two at a time, beating well between additions; add vanilla and allspice, beating well. Add flour mixture a little at a time until well mixed. Turn batter into greased and lightly floured Bundt pan (or two 9″ × 5″ × 3″ bread pans). Bake 1¼ to 1½ hours for Bundt cake or 1 hour for loaf cakes. Cool in pans; turn out on wire rack and cool completely. May be sprinkled with substitute confectioners' sugar.

STRAWBERRY SHORTCAKE

Exchanges per serving: 1 cake = 1½ Starch, ⅔ Fat
½ cup berries = ½ Fruit

Calories per serving: cake, 170   Yield: 6 servings
berries, 30
topping, 14 per tablespoon

2 cups flour
Nonnutritive sweetener
  equivalent to 1
  tablespoon sugar
½ teaspoon salt
3 teaspoons baking
  powder
4 tablespoons diet
  margarine
½ cup water

1 quart strawberries (or
  other fruit) sweetened
  with nonnutritive
  sweetener equivalent to
  1 teaspoon sugar
1 cup nondairy whipped
  topping, whipped with
  nonnutritive sweetener
  equivalent to 1 teaspoon
  sugar

Preheat oven to 475°F. Sift flour, sweetener, salt, and baking powder; add margarine; mix thoroughly with fork. Add water to make soft dough. Roll out on floured board until about ½" thick and cut with large biscuit cutter dipped in flour, or half-fill large greased muffin rings that have been placed on a baking sheet. Bake 10–12 minutes. Split while hot, and fill with crushed sweetened berries. Put on tops; cover with berries and sweetened whipped topping.

MARY'S SPONGE CAKE

Exchanges per serving: 1½" slice = ½ Starch,
                         ¼ Medium-Fat Meat

Calories per serving: 66   Yield: 12 servings

1 cup flour
¼ cup nonfat dry milk
1 teaspoon baking powder
¼ teaspoon salt
3 eggs
Nonnutritive sweetener
    equivalent to 8 teaspoons
    sugar

2 tablespoons fresh orange
    juice
1 teaspoon orange rind,
    grated
½ teaspoon cream of tartar

Preheat oven to 325°F. Sift flour, dry milk, baking powder, and salt together three times; beat 2 whole eggs and 1 yolk at top speed of mixer until quite thick and lemon-colored (about 10 minutes). Reduce speed; add sweetener gradually, then orange juice; increase speed and beat until very light and fluffy (5–6 minutes). Add rind and beat a little more. Beat remaining egg white slightly; add cream of tartar and continue beating until white holds a stiff peak. Let stand while completing next step. Very carefully fold sifted dry ingredients, a small amount at a time, into egg-sweetener mixture, using rubber spatula or wire whip. Fold in single egg white very carefully. Pour at once into 9" tube pan. (If pan has removable bottom, no need to line or grease pan; knife will help loosen cake from bottom. Otherwise, line just the bottom of pan with piece of thin waxed paper, moistened well with water to make it lie flat.) Bake about 35 minutes. Cake is done when it springs back when touched with finger. Cool in pan upside down and remove carefully.

AUNT JEANNE'S SPONGE CAKE

Exchanges per serving: ½″ slice = ½ Starch,
                              ⅓ Medium-Fat Meat
Calories per serving: 70 (does not include ice cream exchange
                        and calorie count)   Yield: 20 servings

1 cup nonfat milk	6 eggs
1¾ cups flour	Nonnutritive sweetener
2 teaspoons baking	equivalent to 2 cups
powder	sugar
½ teaspoon salt	2 teaspoons vanilla

Preheat oven to 350°F. Scald nonfat milk in small saucepan. Remove from heat; put aside until lukewarm. Sift flour, baking powder, and salt. Beat eggs until thick and lemon-colored; gradually add sweetener, beating, until mixture is well blended and smooth (4–5 minutes). Blend in flour mixture at low speed of mixer until smooth; add lukewarm milk and vanilla. Continue beating until well mixed. Pour batter into ungreased 10″ tube pan; bake 50 minutes, or until tester inserted in center of cake comes out clean. Turn cake—and cake pan—upside down; place tube over the neck of a bottle. This allows air to circulate around top (upside down) of cake, cooling it. Serve with imitation strawberry ice cream.

VANILLA SPONGE ROLL

Exchanges per serving: 1 serving = ⅓ Starch,
                              ⅔ Medium-Fat Meat
Calories per serving: 76 + 32 calories for jelly   Yield: 6 servings

4 eggs, separated	1 teaspoon baking powder
Nonnutritive sweetener	5 tablespoons potato flour
equivalent to 4	1 teaspoon vanilla
tablespoons sugar	¼ cup dietetic jelly

Preheat oven to 325°F. Beat egg whites until stiff; add sweetener. Fold in beaten yolks and remaining ingredients (except jelly). Spread in 15″ × 10″ oblong pan lined with paper greased on both sides; bake 40 minutes. Remove from oven and run knife around edge. Turn out onto towel, remove paper carefully; roll up immediately and let stand one minute. Unfold; cool. Spread cake with dietetic jelly, roll, and dust with granulated sugar substitute.

EASY SPONGE CAKE

Exchanges per serving: 1 slice = ¾ Starch, ½ Medium-Fat Meat
Calories per serving: 100   Yield: 8 slices

1 cup egg whites (5–6)	1 cup flour
4 egg yolks	1 teaspoon baking powder
Nonnutritive sweetener	½ teaspoon vanilla or ½
equivalent to 1 cup sugar	teaspoon lemon juice

Preheat oven to 300°F. Beat egg whites very stiff; beat yolks until very light. Add half the sweetener to whites, the rest to yolks. Mix together and beat hard. Sift flour with baking powder; fold into egg mixture. Add vanilla or lemon juice. Pour into angel cake pan; bake 40 minutes, or until tester inserted in center comes out clean.

FRUIT SPONGE CAKE

Exchanges per serving: 1 serving = ⅔ Starch,
⅓ Medium-Fat Meat

Calories per serving: 84   Yield: 12 servings

1 tablespoon fresh orange
  rind, grated
½ cup fresh orange juice
4 eggs, separated
Nonnutritive sweetener
  equivalent to ½ cup
  sugar

2 tablespoons fresh lemon
  juice
½ teaspoon vanilla extract
1½ cups flour
¼ teaspoon salt
¾ teaspoon cream of tartar

Preheat oven to 325°F. Combine rind and juice. Beat egg yolks until thick and lemon-colored, using highest speed of mixer. To juice and rind of orange, add sweetener, lemon juice, and vanilla extract. Sift flour and salt together; beat into egg yolks, alternating with liquid. Beat whites with cream of tartar until stiff peaks form. Fold the batter into the whites, being careful not to beat. Pour into 9″ ungreased tube pan; bake until done (about 1 hour). Invert pan on bottle to cool.

COFFEE SPONGE CAKE

Exchanges per serving: 1 serving = ⅓ Very Lean Meat
Calories per serving: 26   Yield: 10 servings

2 cups nonfat milk
2 tablespoons instant
  coffee
Nonnutritive sweetener
  equivalent to ¾ cup
  sugar

2 envelopes unflavored
  gelatin
6 egg whites

Scald nonfat milk. Dissolve coffee, ⅓ sugar substitute (equivalent to ¼ cup sugar), and gelatin in scalded milk; chill until slightly thickened. Beat four egg whites stiff; fold in coffee mixture. Pour into mold; chill until firm. Beat remaining two egg whites, gradually adding remaining sugar substitute; continue beating until stiff. Spread over mold with spatula, bringing to edges.

POLLY'S DIETETIC JELLY ROLL

Exchanges per serving: 1 serving = ½ Starch,
$\quad\quad\quad\quad\quad\quad\quad\quad\quad\quad\quad$ ¼ Medium-Fat Meat

Calories per serving: 76 $\quad\quad\quad\quad\quad\quad\quad\quad$ Yield: 12 servings

3 eggs, separated	½ teaspoon lemon extract
Nonnutritive sweetener equivalent to ⅓ cup sugar	1 cup flour
	⅓ cup nonfat dry milk
	1 teaspoon baking powder
2 tablespoons orange juice	¼ teaspoon salt
4 teaspoons liquid from any dietetic fruit	½ teaspoon cream of tartar
	½ cup dietetic jelly

Preheat oven to 325°F. Mix egg yolks, sweetener, orange juice, liquid from fruit, and lemon extract. Beat 10 minutes with electric beater until very light and fluffy. Sift flour, dry milk, baking powder, and salt together three times. Very carefully fold sifted dry ingredients into whipped mixture. Beat egg whites and cream of tartar together until mixture stands in soft peaks. Fold into cake mixture. Pour into jelly-roll pan (about 15″ × 10″), which has been lined with lightly greased waxed paper. Bake about 20 minutes; cake will spring back when touched with finger. Remove from oven and run knife around edge. Turn out onto towel, remove paper carefully, and roll up immediately; let stand one minute; unfold to cool. Fill with jelly and reroll. Slice to serve.

NOTE: Jelly roll must be kept in refrigerator. Any dietetic pudding mix may be used for filling. When pudding is set, beat and put in roll.

ORANGE CUPCAKES

Exchanges per serving: 1 cupcake = ⅓ Starch, ¼ Fat
Calories per serving: (does not include frosting) 46   Yield: 30
                                                              cupcakes

½ cup diet margarine
Nonnutritive sweetener
  equivalent to 1 cup sugar
2 eggs, beaten
⅔ cup orange juice,
  strained

¼ teaspoon salt
2 cups flour
2 teaspoons baking
  powder

Preheat oven to 325°F. Cream margarine and sweetener; add
remaining ingredients. Beat one minute or longer in mixer at
high speed. Pour into baking-cup-lined muffin tins. Bake until
brown. Cool and frost, if desired.

CUPCAKES

Exchanges per serving: 1 cupcake = ⅔ Starch, ⅔ Fat, ⅓ Fruit
Calories per serving: 119   Yield: 12 cupcakes

1½ cups flour
1½ teaspoons baking
  powder
½ teaspoon salt
¼ teaspoon baking soda
½ teaspoon cinnamon
½ teaspoon allspice
½ teaspoon nutmeg

¼ teaspoon ground cloves
½ cup diet margarine
2 eggs
Nonnutritive sweetener
  equivalent to ⅔ cup
  sugar
½ cup white raisins
½ cup cold water

Preheat oven to 350°F. Combine flour, baking powder, salt,
baking soda, cinnamon, allspice, nutmeg, and cloves; cut in
margarine until size of small peas. Add remaining ingredients;
mix until entire mixture is moistened. Place 12 paper baking
cups in muffin tin and fill about half full; bake until tester inserted in center comes out clean.

GINGERBREAD

Exchanges per serving: 1 serving = ¾ Starch, ½ Fat
Calories per serving: 83   Yield: 8 servings

4 tablespoons diet margarine	1½ cups plus 1 tablespoon boiling water
2 tablespoons molasses	1 cup rye flour
½ teaspoon ginger	⅛ teaspoon baking powder
¼ teaspoon cinnamon	4 teaspoons baking soda
¼ teaspoon salt	

Preheat oven to 400°F. Measure margarine, molasses, ginger, cinnamon, and salt into bowl; add boiling water. Sift flour, baking powder, and baking soda into mixture; beat. Pour into greased oblong pan (15″ × 10″); bake 30 minutes.

CAKE FILLING

Exchanges per serving: 1 tablespoon = None
Calories per serving: 11   Yield: 1½ cups

1 recipe Lemon Frosting (see following recipe)	1½ teaspoons unflavored gelatin
1 cup low-fat cottage cheese, drained and sieved	2 tablespoons water

To Lemon Frosting, add cottage cheese; beat until smooth. Add gelatin to water and dissolve over boiling water (about 5 minutes). Blend carefully and use at once.

LEMON FROSTING

Exchanges per serving: 1 tablespoon = None
Calories per serving: 7   Yield: ⅓ cup

2 tablespoons nonfat dry milk	1 teaspoon vanilla
1½ tablespoons lemon juice	½ teaspoon unflavored gelatin
Nonnutritive sweetener equivalent to 2 tablespoons sugar	2 tablespoons water

Combine all ingredients except gelatin and water. Dissolve ½ teaspoon gelatin in 2 tablespoons water over hot water. Beat remaining ingredients at high speed of electric mixer about 15 minutes. Add gelatin gradually. Continue beating until frosting stands in peaks. Use immediately.

LOW-CALORIE FROSTING

Exchanges per serving: 1 tablespoon = ⅓ Lean Meat
Calories per serving: 24   Yield: ¾ cup

4-ounce package Neufchâtel cheese	¼ teaspoon salt
4 teaspoons nonfat milk	1 teaspoon vanilla extract
Nonnutritive sweetener equivalent to ½ cup powdered sugar	Food coloring as desired

Cream cheese and nonfat milk thoroughly; add sweetener, salt, and vanilla; blend well. Add coloring last.

NOTE: If you wish to frost more than ½ dozen cupcakes, increase amounts accordingly.

CREAMY FROSTING

Exchanges per serving: 1 tablespoon = None
Calories per serving: 15   Yield: ½ cup

½ cup low-fat cottage
cheese, sieved
⅛ teaspoon salt
½ tablespoon diet
margarine, melted

Nonnutritive sweetener
equivalent to ½ cup
sugar
1 teaspoon almond or
vanilla extract

Mix all ingredients; beat until smooth. Spread on cake. Frosts one 10″ cake.

COOKIES

BROWNIES DIVINE

Exchanges per serving: 1 brownie = ¼ Starch, 1 Fat
Calories per serving: 80   Yield: 16 brownies

½ cup diet margarine
Nonnutritive sweetener
   equivalent to 1¼ cups
   sugar
1 square unsweetened
   chocolate

1 teaspoon vanilla extract
2 eggs
¾ cup flour
1 teaspoon baking powder
½ cup nuts, chopped

Preheat oven to 350°F. Cream margarine and sweetener until light and fluffy. Place chocolate in aluminum foil; melt over boiling water. Stir chocolate into margarine mixture; beat until smooth. Beat in vanilla and eggs. Sift and stir together flour and baking powder; add nuts; stir this mixture into first mixture until smooth. Grease an 8″ square pan; pour in batter; bake until brownies are shiny, about 30 minutes. Cool in pan; cut into 16 pieces. Serve cool.

BROWNIES

Exchanges per serving: 1 brownie = ¼ Starch, ½ Fat
Calories per serving: 60   Yield: 48 brownies

1 cup diet margarine
2 squares unsweetened
   chocolate
2 cups flour
½ teaspoon salt
1 teaspoon baking soda

Nonnutritive sweetener
   equivalent to 2 cups
   sugar
4 eggs, well beaten
1 teaspoon vanilla extract
½ cup nuts, chopped

Preheat oven to 325°F. Melt margarine and chocolate over low heat; set aside. Sift together flour, salt, and baking soda. Add sweetener, eggs, and vanilla to margarine and chocolate; stir into dry ingredients until well blended; stir in nuts. Pour into 13″ × 9″ pan that has been sprayed well with pan coating. Bake 20 minutes; cool. Cut into 1½″ squares.

TASTY DIET BROWNIES

Exchanges per serving: 1 brownie = ¼ Starch, ½ Fat
Calories per serving: 50   Yield: 16 brownies

⅔ cup flour, sifted
½ teaspoon baking powder
¼ teaspoon salt
1 ounce (1 square) unsweetened chocolate
1 egg
½ cup dietetic maple syrup
Nonnutritive sweetener equivalent to 2 teaspoons sugar
⅓ cup walnuts, chopped
½ teaspoon vanilla extract

Preheat oven to 350°F. Measure sifted flour; add baking powder and salt; sift again. Melt chocolate over hot water. Beat egg one minute; add maple syrup and sweetener; beat two more minutes. Add melted chocolate; blend. Add flour mixture and stir (do not beat) until smooth. Add walnuts and vanilla. Spread batter ½″ to ¾″ thick in an 8″ square pan or 9″ pie tin. Bake 40 minutes.

CHOCOLATE BITES

Exchanges per serving: 2 cookies = ⅓ Fat, ⅓ Starch
Calories per serving: 60   Yield: 2½ dozen cookies

⅓ cup diet margarine
¼ cup cocoa
¼ cup liquid artificial sweetener
2 eggs, well beaten
2 teaspoons vanilla extract
1 cup flour
½ teaspoon baking soda
½ teaspoon salt

Preheat oven to 325°F. Melt margarine; add cocoa, sweetener, eggs, and vanilla; stir until well blended. Sift flour, baking soda, and salt together; add and mix well (batter will be quite dry). Spread in well-greased 8″ square pan. Bake about 20 minutes. Cool and cut into bites.

CHOCOLATE COOKIES

Exchanges per serving: 1 cookie, 2" diameter = ¼ Starch
Calories per serving: 24   Yield: 2½ dozen cookies

1 egg, separated	1 cup flour
Nonnutritive sweetener equivalent to ⅓ cup sugar	1 teaspoon baking powder
	¼ teaspoon salt
	½ cup dietetic chocolate topping
2 teaspoons unsweetened fruit liquid, any kind	¼ teaspoon cream of tartar

Preheat oven to 325°F. Mix egg yolk, sweetener, and fruit liquid together in large bowl. Beat with electric mixer until light and fluffy (about 10–12 minutes). Meanwhile, sift flour, baking powder, and salt together three times. Add chocolate topping to liquid mixture; beat until thoroughly mixed. Beat egg white with cream of tartar until it stands in soft peaks. Very carefully fold dry ingredients into chocolate topping mix. Fold beaten egg white into this mixture; drop by teaspoonfuls onto lightly greased cookie sheet. Bake about 10 minutes or until cookie springs back when lightly touched. Remove cookies with spatula to wire rack to cool.

MARY'S CHOCOLATE CHIP COOKIES

Exchanges per serving: 1 cookie = ½ Fat, without nuts
                               = ¾ Fat, with nuts
Calories per serving: without nuts, 40   Yield: 3
                     with nuts, 50   dozen cookies

¼ teaspoon salt	½ teaspoon vanilla extract
½ teaspoon baking soda	1 egg, beaten
1 cup flour, sifted	½ cup semisweet chocolate, shaved fine
½ cup diet margarine	
Nonnutritive sweetener equivalent to ¾ cup sugar	½ cup nuts, if desired

Preheat oven to 375°F. Sift salt, baking soda, and flour together. Cream margarine; add sweetener, vanilla, and egg; blend well. Add flour mixture; beat well. Stir in chocolate; add nuts (if desired). Drop by level spoonfuls onto a lightly greased baking sheet. Bake about 10 minutes.

CRISP APPLESAUCE COOKIES

Exchanges per serving: 1 cookie = ¼ Starch
Calories per serving: 35   Yield: 4 dozen cookies

1⅔ cups flour, sifted
1 teaspoon cinnamon
¼ teaspoon nutmeg
¼ teaspoon cloves
½ teaspoon allspice
½ teaspoon salt
1 teaspoon baking soda
½ cup diet margarine

Nonnutritive sweetener
  equivalent to 1 cup sugar
1 egg
1 cup unsweetened
  applesauce
⅓ cup white raisins
1 cup whole bran cereal

Preheat oven to 375°F. Sift first seven ingredients together. Beat margarine, sweetener, and egg until light and fluffy. Add flour mixture and applesauce alternately; mix well after each addition. Fold in raisins and cereal. Drop by teaspoonfuls onto well-greased cookie sheet, about 1″ apart. Bake until golden brown (about 15 minutes).

REFRIGERATED COCONUT COOKIES

Exchanges per serving: 2 cookies = ⅓ Starch, ⅓ Fat
Calories per serving: 44　　　　　　　Yield: 2½ dozen cookies,
　　　　　　　　　　　　　　　　　　　　　　¼″ thick each

Nonnutritive sweetener
  equivalent to ½ cup
  sugar
¼ cup unsweetened fruit
  juice
1 teaspoon vanilla extract

¼ teaspoon baking powder
¼ teaspoon salt
1 cup flour
¼ cup diet margarine
2 tablespoons coconut

Preheat oven to 400°F. Combine sweetener, juice, and vanilla extract. Sift together baking powder, salt, and flour; cut in margarine. Add liquid ingredients. After these are well mixed, work in coconut. Form dough into a roll about 7½″ long, 2″ in diameter; wrap in waxed paper and place in refrigerator until well chilled and firm. Slice into thirty ¼″-thick cookies; place on ungreased cookie sheet. Bake 10 minutes.

COCONUT FRUIT COOKIES

Exchanges per serving: 1 cookie = ¼ Starch, ¼ Fat
Calories per serving: 30　　　　　　　Yield: 3 dozen cookies

1½ cups flour
1 teaspoon baking powder
¼ teaspoon baking soda
¼ teaspoon salt
⅓ cup diet margarine
⅓ cup flaked coconut
1 egg
½ cup unsweetened fruit
  juice

2 teaspoons orange or
  lemon peel, grated
Nonnutritive sweetener
  equivalent to ⅓ cup
  sugar
1 teaspoon almond or
  vanilla extract

Preheat oven to 400°F. Combine flour, baking powder, baking soda, and salt; cut in margarine until consistency of peas. Stir in coconut; add remaining ingredients all at once. Stir with fork until dough holds together. Drop about 2″ apart by teaspoonfuls onto an ungreased cookie sheet. Bake until light golden brown (about 10 minutes).

FRUIT COOKIES

Exchanges per serving: 1 cookie = ⅓ Starch, ½ Fat, ¼ Fruit
Calories per serving: 60   Yield: 20 cookies

½ cup flour
⅛ teaspoon cloves
¼ teaspoon nutmeg
1 teaspoon cinnamon
¼ teaspoon salt
½ teaspoon baking soda
½ cup raisins

½ cup rolled oats, uncooked
½ cup dietetic cranberry sauce
½ cup diet margarine, melted
1 egg
1 teaspoon vanilla extract

Preheat oven to 375°F. Sift flour, cloves, nutmeg, cinnamon, salt, and baking soda together; add raisins and oats. Combine cranberry sauce, margarine, egg, and vanilla extract. Stir into dry ingredients until they are moistened. Drop by teaspoonfuls onto lightly greased cookie sheet; bake 10–12 minutes.

SPICY APPLESAUCE COOKIES

Exchanges per serving: two 2″-diameter cookies = ¼ Starch
Calories per serving: 20   Yield: 3½ dozen cookies

1 cup flour	Nonnutritive sweetener
⅓ cup nonfat dry milk	equivalent to 8 teaspoons
1 teaspoon baking powder	sugar
½ teaspoon cinnamon	3 tablespoons unsweetened
¼ teaspoon nutmeg	fruit liquid (any fruit)
¼ teaspoon cloves	½ cup unsweetened
⅛ teaspoon salt	applesauce
2 eggs	10 almonds blanched and
	cut in quarters

Preheat oven to 325°F. Sift dry ingredients together three times. Mix eggs, sweetener, and fruit liquid. Beat at top speed of mixer until fluffy and thick (about 10 minutes). Decrease speed; add applesauce and beat 3 minutes. Carefully fold in dry ingredients. Drop by teaspoonfuls onto lightly greased cookie sheet. Place ¼ almond on each cookie. Bake about 10 minutes. Cookie will spring back at light touch when done. (These may be placed under broiler to give deeper finish.)

ORANGE COOKIES WITH NUTS

Exchanges per serving: 2 cookies = ⅓ Starch, ½ Fat
Calories per serving: 38   Yield: 2½ dozen cookies

½ cup frozen unsweetened	1 cup flour
orange juice concentrate	¼ teaspoon salt
1 egg	¼ teaspoon baking powder
¼ cup diet margarine	1 teaspoon vanilla extract
Nonnutritive sweetener	½ cup pecans, chopped
equivalent to 1 cup sugar	fine

Preheat oven to 375°F. Cream first four ingredients; beat well. Sift flour, salt, and baking powder; add to creamed mixture. Mix gently until just blended; add vanilla and nuts. Drop by teaspoonfuls onto lightly greased cookie sheet; bake until lightly browned (about 15 minutes).

ORANGE (OR LEMON) PEEL COOKIES

Exchanges per serving: 2 cookies = ½ Starch, ¾ Fat
Calories per serving: 73   Yield: 3 dozen cookies

½ cup diet margarine	2 cups flour
Nonnutritive sweetener equivalent to ½ cup sugar	1 teaspoon baking powder
	½ teaspoon salt
⅓ cup hot water	¾ cup pecans, chopped fine
1 teaspoon orange extract	1 tablespoon orange or lemon peel, finely grated
1 teaspoon vanilla extract	

Preheat oven to 400°F. Cream first five ingredients; sift together and add flour, baking powder, and salt. Blend in pecans and orange or lemon peel until mixture is smooth. Shape dough into roll about 2″ × 6″. Wrap in waxed paper; chill well in refrigerator. Cut roll into 36 cookies; place on lightly greased cookie sheet. Bake until brown around edges, about 12–15 minutes.

YUMMY PEANUT BUTTER COOKIES

Exchanges per serving: 1 cookie = ¼ Starch, ½ Fat
Calories per serving: 45   Yield: 18 cookies

⅓ cup flour
¼ teaspoon baking soda
¼ teaspoon baking powder
¼ cup diet margarine
4 tablespoons peanut
   butter

Nonnutritive sweetener
   equivalent to 1
   tablespoon brown sugar
Nonnutritive sweetener
   equivalent to ½ cup
   sugar
1 egg, well beaten

Preheat oven to 375°F. Grease cookie sheet lightly. Sift flour, baking soda, and baking powder. Work margarine and peanut butter with spoon until creamy; gradually add brown sugar substitute; continue working until light. Add regular sugar substitute and egg; beat well. Mix in dry ingredients thoroughly. Drop by teaspoonfuls onto lightly greased cookie sheet; flatten with tines of fork. Bake until done (about 8–10 minutes).

PEANUT BUTTER COOKIES

Exchanges per serving: 1 cookie = ⅓ Starch, ½ Fat
Calories per serving: 80   Yield: 8 cookies

8 graham cracker squares,
   crushed
2 tablespoons peanut
   butter

Nonnutritive sweetener
   equivalent to ¼ cup
   sugar
1 teaspoon baking powder
3 egg yolks
1 teaspoon nonfat milk

Preheat oven to 350°F. Combine graham cracker crumbs and peanut butter; add sweetener and baking powder. Add egg yolks and milk; mix well. Divide into eight 1″ cookies and press with tines of fork to flatten. Bake 10 minutes.

JOAN'S PEANUT BUTTER COOKIES

Exchanges per serving: 5 cookies = ½ Starch, 1¼ Fat,
                                    ½ High-Fat Meat
Calories per serving: 155   Yield: 4 dozen cookies

¼ cup diet margarine	⅓ cup nonfat milk
Nonnutritive sweetener equivalent to 1 cup sugar	1 teaspoon vanilla extract
	1 cup flour
½ cup peanut butter, softened*	¼ teaspoon salt
	1 teaspoon baking powder
1 egg	

Preheat oven to 375°F. Combine margarine, sweetener, and peanut butter and blend well. Combine egg, nonfat milk, and vanilla; add to first mixture. Sift flour, salt, and baking powder together; add, blending well. Drop by spoonfuls onto greased cookie sheet. Flatten with tines of fork dipped in water. Bake 10 minutes.

ANGEL'S KISS

Exchanges per serving: 1 kiss = ¼ Fat, ¼ Medium-Fat Meat
Calories per serving: 26   Yield: 3 dozen kisses

Nonnutritive sweetener equivalent to 1½ cups confectioner's sugar	½ cup blanched almonds, finely cut
1½ cups egg yolks, beaten	1 teaspoon instant diet tea mix
	1 teaspoon almond extract

Preheat oven to 325°F. Beat sweetener into yolks; add almonds, tea mix, and almond extract. Line muffin pans with paper baking cups; fill each half full. Bake until golden brown; remove cups while warm. Cool on wire rack.

* Leave at room temperature until sufficiently soft.

BUTTERMILK OAT COOKIES

Exchanges per serving: 1 square = ¼ Starch
Calories per serving: 29   Yield: 2½ dozen cookies

1 cup flour
¼ teaspoon baking soda
½ teaspoon salt
½ cup rolled oats,
   uncooked

Nonnutritive sweetener
   equivalent to 3
   tablespoons sugar
¼ cup buttermilk
¼ cup diet margarine,
   melted

Preheat oven to 400°F. Sift flour, baking soda, and salt; add oats. Add sweetener to buttermilk; stir with margarine into flour mixture until dry ingredients are moistened. Knead dough lightly on well-floured board for a few minutes; roll thin. Cut into 2″ squares. Bake on ungreased cookie sheet until brown (10–12 minutes).

GRANDMA'S COOKIES

Exchanges per serving: 1 cookie = ½ Starch, ½ Fat
Calories per serving: 57   Yield: 2 dozen cookies

⅔ cup diet margarine
Nonnutritive sweetener
   equivalent to ¾ cup
   sugar
1 teaspoon vanilla extract
1 egg

4 teaspoons nonfat milk
2 cups all-purpose flour,
   sifted
1½ teaspoons baking
   powder
¼ teaspoon salt

Preheat oven to 375°F. Thoroughly cream margarine, sweetener, and vanilla. Add egg; beat until light and fluffy; stir in milk. Sift flour, baking powder, and salt together; blend into creamed mixture. Divide dough in half; chill 1 hour. Roll half of the dough at a time. (Keep balance chilled for easier rolling.) On lightly floured surface, roll dough to about ½″ thickness. Cut in desired shapes; bake 6–8 minutes. Cool slightly, remove from pan. Top each with unsweetened fruit, if desired (some fruit doesn't bake well and will brown). (See Fruit Exchange List for additional calorie count.)

BUTTERSCOTCH SQUARES

Exchanges per serving: 1 square = ¼ Fat

Calories per serving: 25   Yield: 70 squares

½ cup diet margarine	1½ cups flour
Nonnutritive sweetener equivalent to 2 cups brown sugar	2 teaspoons baking powder
2 eggs	1 teaspoon vanilla extract
	½ cup walnuts, chopped

Preheat oven to 350°F. Cook margarine and sweetener together until smooth. Cool to lukewarm. Add eggs; beat well. Add flour, baking powder, vanilla, and walnuts. Spread in lightly greased 13″ × 9″ pan. Bake 30 minutes. Cut into 1¼″ squares. Sprinkle with nonnutritive granulated sugar substitute. Cool.

CREAM CHEESE DELIGHT

Exchanges per serving: 1 cookie = ¼ Starch, ¼ Fat
Calories per serving: 38   Yield: 36 cookies

½ cup diet margarine
3 ounces Neufchâtel
  cheese
Nonnutritive sweetener
  equivalent to ⅓ cup
  sugar
1 egg yolk

1 teaspoon orange extract
1 teaspoon orange rind,
  grated
1 teaspoon lemon rind,
  grated
1½ cups flour, sifted
½ teaspoon salt

Preheat oven to 400°F. Cream softened margarine and cream cheese; add sugar substitute gradually and continue to cream until light and fluffy. Add egg yolk, extract, and rinds; beat well. Add flour and salt, which have been sifted together, to creamed mixture, a little at a time. Chill about 1 hour. Form into small balls; flatten with back of fork tines on ungreased cookie sheet. Bake until brown (10–12 minutes).

MACAROONS

Exchanges per serving: 1 macaroon = ½ Fat
Calories per serving: 24   Yield: 3½ dozen macaroons

1 egg, separated
Nonnutritive sweetener
  equivalent to 1 cup sugar
2 cups cornflakes

1 cup shredded coconut
½ cup chopped pecans
  (optional)
½ teaspoon almond extract

Preheat oven to 350°F. Beat egg white stiff but not dry; fold in sweetener. Add cornflakes, coconut, chopped pecans, and almond extract. Drop from teaspoon onto greased baking sheet; bake about 12 minutes. Remove at once from baking sheet.

SPICY COOKIES

Exchanges per serving: 1 cookie = ¼ Starch, ¼ Fat
Calories per serving: 30   Yield: 24 cookies

⅓ cup diet margarine
1 cup flour
¼ teaspoon baking powder
¼ teaspoon salt
2 tablespoons cocoa
1 tablespoon water

Nonnutritive sweetener
  equivalent to ⅓ cup
  sugar
½ teaspoon cinnamon
½ teaspoon nutmeg
1 teaspoon vanilla extract

Preheat oven to 375°F. Cream margarine until light and nearly cream-colored. Sift flour, baking powder, salt, and cocoa together; blend into margarine until smooth. Mix water, sweetener, cinnamon, nutmeg, and vanilla extract; add to flour-margarine mixture; mix until smooth (dough will be stiff). Shape into balls about ¾″ round. Place on cookie sheet; flatten with blade of knife dipped in cold water. Bake until done (about 15 minutes). Remove from tray and cool.

MARY'S THUMBPRINTS

Exchanges per serving: 1 cookie = ⅓ Fat
Calories per serving: 28   Yield: 4 dozen cookies
plus diet jelly (2 teaspoons = 16 calories)

½ cup diet margarine	½ teaspoon vanilla extract
Nonnutritive sweetener equivalent to ¼ cup sugar	1 tablespoon lemon juice
	1 tablespoon orange juice
1 tablespoon orange rind, grated	1 cup flour
	1 teaspoon salt
1½ teaspoons lemon rind, grated	1 egg, separated
	½ cup nuts, finely chopped
	Diet jelly

Preheat oven to 350°F. Mix together all ingredients except egg whites, nuts, and jelly. Roll into small balls. Beat egg white stiff. Spread the nuts out on a piece of waxed paper. Roll each ball in egg white, then in nuts. Place on cookie sheet and make a thumbprint in each. Bake 12 minutes; cool. When cool, fill each thumbprint with diet jelly.

OATMEAL COOKIES

Exchanges per serving: 1 cookie = ⅓ Starch, ¼ Fat
Calories per serving: 42   Yield: 4 dozen cookies

1½ cups quick-cooking or instant oatmeal, uncooked	1½ cups flour, sifted
	1 teaspoon baking powder
	½ teaspoon salt
⅔ cup diet margarine, melted	½ cup nonfat milk
	1 teaspoon vanilla extract
2 eggs, beaten	¼ cup raisins
Nonnutritive sweetener equivalent to 1½ cups sugar	

Preheat oven to 400°F. Measure oatmeal into bowl; stir in melted margarine; mix well. Stir in eggs and sweetener; add mixture of flour, baking powder, and salt alternately with the combined milk and vanilla. Add raisins. Drop onto cookie sheet from level teaspoon; bake until golden brown (about 10–15 minutes).

RICE FLOUR COOKIES

Exchanges per serving: 1 cookie = ½ Starch, ½ Fat
Calories per serving: 70   Yield: 2 dozen cookies

¾ cup diet margarine
Nonnutritive sweetener
  equivalent to 1½ cups
  sugar
2 eggs
½ teaspoon vanilla extract

½ teaspoon almond extract
1 teaspoon orange or
  lemon extract
2½ cups rice flour
1 teaspoon cream of tartar
1 teaspoon baking soda

Preheat oven to 375°F. Cream margarine and sweetener; add eggs and extracts. Sift flour, cream of tartar, and baking soda; mix all ingredients well; roll into small balls. Place on greased cookie sheet; flatten with tines of fork. Bake until brown (10 minutes).

PIES AND PIECRUSTS

APPLE PIE

Exchanges per serving: 1 filling = ¾ Fruit, ¼ Fat
1 pastry = 1½ Starch, 1½ Fat
Calories per serving: filling, 64   Yield: 8 servings
pastry, 190

Nonnutritive sweetener
  equivalent to ¾ cup
  sugar
2 tablespoons flour
½ teaspoon cinnamon
Dash of nutmeg
Dash of salt
3 cups tart apples, pared,
  cored, and thinly sliced
Pastry for 2-crust 9″ pie
2 tablespoons diet
  margarine

Preheat oven to 400°F. Combine sweetener, flour, spices, and salt; mix with apples. Line pie plate with pastry; fill with apple mixture; dot with margarine. Place top crust on pie: sprinkle with sugar substitute, if desired. Bake about 50 minutes, or until done.

DEEP-DISH APPLE PIE

Exchanges per serving: 1 serving = ¾ Starch, ¾ Fat, ½ Fruit
Calories per serving: 113   Yield: 8 servings

4 apples, pared and sliced
  thin
2 teaspoons lemon juice
½ teaspoon lemon rind,
  grated
¼ teaspoon nutmeg
½ teaspoon cinnamon
Nonnutritive sweetener
  equivalent to 1 cup sugar
½ tablespoon arrowroot
1⅛ teaspoons salt
1 cup flour, sifted
⅓ cup diet margarine
⅓ cup water

Preheat oven to 425°F. Combine apples, lemon juice, lemon rind, nutmeg, cinnamon, sweetener, arrowroot, and ⅛ teaspoon salt. Pour into well-buttered 9″ deep-dish pie plate. Combine flour and 1 teaspoon salt; cut in margarine until consistency of cornmeal; blend in water; roll out as for a piecrust; place on top of filling. Bake until crust is brown (about 35 minutes).

MYRA'S APPLE PIE

Exchanges per serving: 1 serving = 1 Starch, 1 Fat, 1 Fruit
Calories per serving: 189   Yield: 12 servings

2 cups flour	3 tablespoons lemon juice
Nonnutritive sweetener equivalent to 1⅓ cups sugar	1 cup water 10 apples, peeled, cored, and sliced
¾ cup diet margarine	½ cup white raisins
1 egg	1 teaspoon cinnamon

Preheat oven to 375°F. Mix flour with about ⅔ of the sweetener; crumble margarine into flour mixture with fingers until mixture is size of peas. Stir in egg with fork until well blended. Work dough with hands until a smooth ball; divide into 3 sections. Wrap ⅓ dough in waxed paper; store in refrigerator until ready for top crust. Grease a 10″ springform pan lightly; press remaining ⅔ dough firmly and evenly over bottom and about ¾ up the sides of pan; set aside. Mix lemon juice and water; add apples a few at a time to the lemon-water to moisten each slice thoroughly. When apples are moistened, squeeze moisture out with hands and place apples in large bowl. Add raisins, balance of sweetener, and cinnamon. Stir and mix. Place in crust. Roll refrigerated ⅓ dough on well-floured board, to 1″ larger than pan. Fit dough over apples, pressing side and top together with wet fingers (so surface is flush with top). Prick pastry with fork several times; bake 1 hour and 10 minutes. Cool 10 minutes; loosen but leave in pan until room temperature.

GREAT APPLE AND GRAPE PIE

Exchanges per serving: 1 filling = 1½ Fruit
                     1 pastry = 1 Starch, 1 Fat
Calories per serving: filling, 100   Yield: 6 servings
                    pastry, 120

3 tablespoons tapioca	½ cup water
Dash of salt	Nonnutritive sweetener
3 cups apples, cored,	equivalent to 1 cup sugar
pared, and sliced	2 tablespoons lemon juice
2 cups seedless grapes, cut	1 tablespoon diet
in halves	margarine, melted
Pastry for one 9″ piecrust,	
unbaked (see Index)	

Preheat oven to 425°F. Mix tapioca and salt; toss with apples and grapes. Place in unbaked pie shell. Combine remaining ingredients; pour over fruit. Cover top with aluminum foil; bake 15 minutes. Reduce heat to 325°F, and continue baking until apples are tender (about 50 minutes).

QUICK APPLE PIE

Exchanges per serving: 1 filling = 1 Fruit
                     1 pastry = 1½ Starch, 3 Fat
Calories per serving: filling, 60   Yield: 8 servings
                    pastry, 250

4 cups apples, pared, cored,	½ teaspoon cinnamon
sliced very thin	1 tablespoon arrowroot
2 teaspoons lemon juice	Nonnutritive sweetener
¼ teaspoon lemon peel,	equivalent to ¾ cup sugar
finely grated	1 recipe Rich Flaky Crust
¼ teaspoon nutmeg	(see Index)

Preheat oven to 425°F. Mix together all ingredients except pastry. Prepare crust, lining an 8″ pie plate. Fill with apple mixture and top with second crust; flute edges. Make 4 or 5 cuts for air vents. Lightly cover fluted edges with aluminum foil to prevent excessive browning of crust. After about 30 minutes, remove foil and continue baking until apples are tender (another 10–20 minutes). Cool.

SHERRY'S APPLE PIE

Exchanges per serving: 1 filling = 1 Fruit
1 pastry = 2 Starch, 2 Fat
Calories per serving: filling, 60   Yield: 6 servings
pastry, 240

Pastry for 2-crust 9″ pie (see Index)
5 apples, sliced
2 teaspoons tapioca
Nonnutritive sweetener equivalent to ½ cup sugar
Dash of cinnamon

Preheat oven to 400°F. Roll ½ crust recipe to fit a 9″ pie pan; arrange apple slices in crust; sprinkle tapioca, sweetener, and cinnamon over top. Roll out remaining crust; crimp edges securely over top (moisten edges between crusts with water if necessary); perforate in about six places. Bake until apples are tender (about 30 minutes).

NOTE: If a 1-crust pie is desired, adjust exchanges per serving to 1 Starch, 1 Fat, and subtract 120 calories per serving.

JIFFY BANANA CREAM PIE

Exchanges per serving: 1 filling = ¼ Fruit, ¼ Nonfat Milk
1 pastry = ¾ Starch, ¾ Fat
Calories per serving: filling, 80   Yield: 8 servings
pastry, 95

2 packages dietetic vanilla pudding mix
2 cups nonfat milk
2 bananas, sliced (or other fruit, such as peaches, strawberries)
8″ baked pastry (see Index)

Prepare pudding mix, using nonfat milk; cool slightly. Cover bottom of pie shell with banana slices. Fill with pudding and let stand until set.

BERRY PIE

Exchanges per serving: 1 filling = ½ Fruit
1 pastry = 1 Starch, 1 Fat
Calories per serving: filling, 20   Yield: 8 servings
pastry, 120

1 quart berries (e.g., blueberries, raspberries)	1 tablespoon arrowroot
2 teaspoons lemon juice	Nonnutritive sweetener equivalent to ¾ cup sugar
¼ teaspoon lemon peel, finely grated	Pastry for one 9″ piecrust, unbaked (see Index)
½ teaspoon cinnamon	

Preheat oven to 425°F. Wash berries; mix with next five ingredients. Put into piecrust; bake until tender (45–50 minutes). If a 2-crust pie is desired, cover pie before baking, cut vents in the top crust, flute edges, and cover fluting with aluminum foil to prevent excessive browning.

NOTE: For a 2-crust pie, adjust exchanges per serving to 2 Starch, 2 Fat, and add an additional 120 calories.

BANANA CREAM PIE

Exchanges per serving: 1 filling = ¼ Skim Milk
1 pastry = 1 Starch, 1 Fat
Calories per serving: filling, 60   Yield: 6 servings
pastry, 120

Pastry for one 9″ piecrust (see Index)	Nonnutritive sweetener equivalent to ½ cup sugar
¼ cup flour	⅛ teaspoon salt
1½ cups nonfat milk	1 medium banana
1 egg, beaten	Nondairy whipped topping (optional) 10–15 calories per tablespoon
1 teaspoon lemon juice	
½ teaspoon vanilla extract	

Bake and cool pie shell. Blend flour with ½ cup cold nonfat milk. Scald remaining 1 cup nonfat milk; add flour-milk mixture and egg, lemon juice, vanilla, sweetener, and salt. Cook in top of double boiler, stirring until thick. Slice banana into pie shell. Spread cream filling over top; cool. Cover with nondairy whipped topping, if desired. Serve immediately.

CHIFFON EGGNOG PIE

Exchanges per serving: 1 filling = ⅓ Medium-Fat Meat,
¼ Skim Milk
1 pastry = 1 Starch, 1 Fat
Calories per serving: filling, 57   Yield: 6 servings
pastry, 120

1 envelope unflavored gelatin	¼ teaspoon salt
¼ cup cold water	½ tablespoon arrowroot
1½ cups nonfat milk	2 eggs, separated
Nonnutritive sweetener equivalent to ¾ cup sugar	1 teaspoon almond extract
	1 tablespoon rum extract
	9″ baked piecrust (see Index)

Soften gelatin in cold water. Combine ¾ cup nonfat milk, sweetener, and salt in top of double boiler. Make a paste of arrowroot and remaining milk; stir into first mixture. Cook over boiling water, stirring constantly until thick. Beat egg yolks and add a little of the hot mixture; stir into remaining hot liquid in double boiler. Cook another 2 minutes; remove from heat; stir in softened gelatin until dissolved. Chill until mixture begins to set; stir in extracts. Beat egg whites very stiff; fold into gelatin mixture. Pour into baked pie shell; chill until firm. If desired, top with Low-Calorie Topping Whip (see Index) or artificial whipped cream; sprinkle chocolate shavings over this.

NOTE: Add additional calories and exchanges if Low-Calorie Topping Whip is used.

ICEBOX CHOCOLATE PIE

Exchanges per serving: 1 serving = ½ Starch
Calories per serving: 68   Yield: 8 servings

2 tablespoons cocoa
⅛ teaspoon salt
1½ teaspoons arrowroot
½ cup nonfat milk, scalded
1 egg, separated

Nonnutritive sweetener
   equivalent to ¾ cup
   sugar
½ cup evaporated milk,
   beaten
1 teaspoon vanilla
12 graham cracker squares

Mix cocoa, salt, and arrowroot; blend in nonfat milk. Add slightly beaten egg yolk and sweetener; cook in top of double boiler until thickened; cool. Beat egg white, evaporated milk, and vanilla until stiff; fold into first mixture. Roll graham crackers into crumbs; sprinkle half in 8″ pie pan; pour in filling. Sprinkle remaining crumbs on top. Put in freezer until firm.

PEACHY PIE

Exchanges per serving: 1 serving = ⅓ Starch, 1⅓ Fruit
Calories per serving: 110   Yield: 6 servings

1½ cups cornflakes
1 tablespoon diet
   margarine, melted
1 teaspoon hot water
4 cups unsweetened
   canned or fresh peaches,
   sliced*
2 envelopes dietetic cherry
   gelatin

1 tablespoon lemon juice
1 teaspoon lemon rind,
   grated
¼ cup nonfat dry milk
¼ cup cold water
Nonnutritive sweetener
   equivalent to 3
   tablespoons sugar

Preheat oven to 325°F. Crush cornflakes. Mix margarine and hot water; add to cornflakes; mix thoroughly. Spread mixture evenly in an 8″ pie pan; press firmly around edge with spatula.

* If using fresh peaches, use 1 cup water in lieu of juice.

Bake 8–10 minutes; cool. Drain peaches, reserving juice; add water to make 1 cup liquid. Dissolve gelatin in liquid. Heat almost to boiling; add 2 teaspoons lemon juice and rind; cool. Chop and add peaches; chill until mixture begins to thicken. Mix nonfat dry milk, cold water, and remaining lemon juice; whip until mixture stands in peaks. Add sweetener; beat until mixture stands in very stiff peaks. Very carefully fold gelatin-peach mixture into whipped milk; mix. Pour gently into pie shell; serve chilled.

PEACH PIE

Exchanges per serving: 1 filling = ½ Fruit
 1 pastry = 1 Starch, 1½ Fat
Calories per serving: filling, 26   Yield: 10 servings
 pastry, 130

2 cups firm, ripe peaches
¼ tablespoon salt
Water
Nonnutritive sweetener
 equivalent to ½ cup
 sugar

¼ teaspoon lemon juice
Pastry for one 9″ piecrust,
 unbaked
2 tablespoons diet
 margarine

Preheat oven to 325°F. Peel and pit peaches; slice and drop into solution of salt and 1 quart hot water; drain. Mix sweetener, ¼ cup water, and lemon juice together; pour over peaches. Set in refrigerator until cool. Place in unbaked 9″ piecrust; dot with margarine. Bake until peaches are tender to the touch of a fork (30–40 minutes).

PEACH COBBLER

Exchanges per serving: 1 serving = ⅓ Starch, ½ Fruit
Calories per serving: 78 per ⅛ cobbler   Yield: 8 servings

4 fresh peaches, peeled and
  cut into ⅛" slices
1 tablespoon lemon juice
1 teaspoon lemon rind,
  finely grated
1 tablespoon arrowroot
1 tablespoon allspice

¼ teaspoon salt
Nonnutritive sweetener
  equivalent to ½ cup
  sugar
½ cup flour
3 tablespoons diet
  margarine

Preheat oven to 425°F. Spray pie plate with Pam or other nonfat spray. Combine peaches, lemon juice, and lemon rind in large mixing bowl. Combine arrowroot, allspice, ½ the salt, and the sweetener; mix well. Place over peaches and shake bowl gently to coat all pieces of fruit; spread peaches evenly in pie plate. Make crumb mixture of flour, remaining salt, and diet margarine; spread evenly over top of peaches. Bake until crumbs are nicely browned, 35–40 minutes. Serve hot.

CHIFFON PUMPKIN PIE

Exchanges per serving: 1 filling = ½ Medium-Fat Meat,
                                    ¼ Skim Milk, ½ Starch
                        1 pastry = 1 Starch, 1 Fat
Calories per serving: filling, 93   Yield: 8 servings
                      pastry, 120

Pastry for one 9" piecrust
  (see Index)
1 envelope unflavored
  gelatin
1 cup evaporated milk
½ cup water
½ teaspoon nutmeg
½ teaspoon cinnamon

¼ teaspoon ginger
½ teaspoon salt
4 eggs, separated
Nonnutritive sweetener
  equivalent to ¾ cup
  sugar
1¼ cups canned pumpkin,
  mashed

Line a 9″ pie plate with desired crust. Bake and cool. Combine next eight ingredients, reserving egg whites; beat well. Stir and cook in top of double boiler until consistency of medium white sauce (about 10 minutes). Stir in sweetener. Place in refrigerator until cold. Beat whites until they form soft peaks. Fold pumpkin into gelatin mixture; add beaten egg whites carefully; pour into pie shell and chill until set.

OLGA'S PUMPKIN PIE

Exchanges per serving: 1 serving = 1½ Starch
Calories per serving: 110   Yield: 6 servings

1½ cups cornflakes	2 envelopes dietetic
1 teaspoon diet margarine, melted	butterscotch or vanilla pudding
1 tablespoon hot water	1 cup pumpkin, canned or
½ cup dietetic maple syrup	fresh cooked
1 cup nonfat milk	1 egg

Preheat oven to 325°F. Crush cornflakes. Mix margarine and water; add to cornflakes; mix thoroughly. Spread mixture evenly in a 9″ pie pan; press firmly around edge with spatula. Bake 8–10 minutes; cool. Blend remaining ingredients in saucepan; cook over medium heat, stirring constantly until mixture comes to a boil. Cool to room temperature; pour into pie shell. Chill at least three hours before serving.

PUMPKIN PIE

Exchanges per serving: 1 filling = ¼ Medium-Fat Meat,
¾ Skim Milk, ⅓ Starch
1 pastry = 1 Starch, 1 Fat
Calories per serving: filling, 135   Yield: 8 servings
pastry, 120

1½ cups canned or fresh
cooked pumpkin
Nonnutritive sweetener
equivalent to ¾ cup
sugar
½ teaspoon salt
1¼ teaspoons cinnamon
½–1 teaspoon ginger

¼–½ teaspoon nutmeg
¼–½ teaspoon cloves
2 eggs, slightly beaten
1¼ cups nonfat milk
2 cups nonfat evaporated
milk
Pastry for one 9″ piecrust,
unbaked (see Index)

Preheat oven to 400°F. Combine pumpkin, sweetener, salt, and spices thoroughly; blend in eggs, milk, and evaporated milk. Pour into unbaked pastry shell; bake until knife inserted between center and outside comes out clean. Serve cool.

MARY C'S PUMPKIN PIE

Exchanges per serving: 1 filling = ¼ Nonfat Milk, ½ Starch,
¼ Fruit
1 pastry = 1 Starch, 1 Fat
Calories per serving: filling, 90   Yield: 6 servings
pastry, 120

1 egg
Nonnutritive sweetener
equivalent to 1 cup sugar
¾ teaspoon allspice
¾ teaspoon nutmeg
¾ teaspoon cinnamon

½ teaspoon ginger
¼ teaspoon cloves
1½ cups canned pumpkin
¾ cup evaporated milk
¾ cup fresh orange juice
One 9″ piecrust, unbaked

Preheat oven to 425°F. Combine egg, sweetener, spices, and pumpkin; blend well. Add milk and orange juice gradually; stir until well blended. Pour into unbaked pie shell; bake 10–12 minutes, then reduce heat to 325°F; bake until a knife inserted near center comes out clean (about 45 minutes).

POLLY'S PUMPKIN PIE

Exchanges per serving: 1 filling = ¼ Medium-Fat Meat,
                                   ½ Skim Milk, ⅓ Starch
                       1 pastry = 1 Starch, 1 Fat
Calories per serving: filling, 90   Yield: 8 servings
                      pastry, 120

Nonnutritive sweetener equivalent to 1 cup sugar	½ teaspoon cloves
1½ teaspoons cinnamon	1¾ cups evaporated milk
½ teaspoon allspice	2 eggs, well beaten
½ teaspoon ginger	1½ cups canned pumpkin
½ teaspoon nutmeg	One 9″ unbaked pie shell, chilled (see Index)

Preheat oven to 425°F. Combine sweetener and spices; stir in evaporated milk and eggs; add pumpkin. Beat until smooth. Pour mixture into a chilled 9″ pie shell (do not prick bottom of shell). Bake at 425°F for 15 minutes, then reduce heat to 350°F; bake until knife inserted in center of pie comes out clean (about 35–40 minutes). Cool.

FRUIT FILLING FOR PIE

Exchanges per serving: 1 filling = 1 Fruit
1 pastry = 1 Starch, 1 Fat
Calories per serving: filling, 60   Yield: 8 servings
pastry, 120

4 cups any fruit (apples, blueberries, fresh peaches, pears, orange sections, pineapple, seedless grapes, etc.)	1 tablespoon arrowroot
	¼ teaspoon lemon peel, grated fine
	2 teaspoons lemon juice
Nonnutritive sweetener equivalent to ¾ cup sugar	¼ teaspoon nutmeg
	½ teaspoon cinnamon
	Pastry for one 9″ piecrust, unbaked (see Index)

Preheat oven to 425°F. Mix all ingredients together and place in piecrust. Bake until fruit is tender (about 45–50 minutes). If a 2-crust pie is desired, cover unbaked pie with second crust, cut air vents in top, and flute edges. Cover fluted edges with foil to prevent excessive browning (remove foil after 30 minutes), and bake as before.

NOTE: For a 2-crust pie, adjust exchanges per serving to 2 Starch, 2 Fat, and pastry calories to 240.

RICE CEREAL PIECRUST

Exchanges per serving: 1 serving = ¼ Fat, ⅛ Starch
Calories per serving: 18   Yield: one 8″ crust

1 cup crispy rice cereal, crushed	Nonnutritive sweetener equivalent to 4 tablespoons sugar
2 tablespoons diet margarine, melted	

Mix ingredients together; line bottom and sides of 8″ pan; chill well before adding any desired filling.

FRUIT COBBLER

Exchanges per serving: 1 serving = ¾ Starch, ¼ Fruit,
                                   ¼ Medium-Fat Meat, ¼ Fat
Calories per serving: 155   Yield: 4 servings

2 cups water-packed fruit (e.g., cherries), unsweetened; reserve juice	⅛ teaspoon salt
	¾ teaspoon baking powder
	1 tablespoon diet margarine
¼ teaspoon lemon juice	1 egg
⅛ teaspoon almond extract	2 tablespoons nonfat milk
½ teaspoon arrowroot	Nonnutritive sweetener equivalent to ¼ cup sugar
⅔ cup juice from fruit	
½ cup flour, sifted	

Preheat oven to 425°F. Place a layer of drained fruit in a shallow cake pan. Combine lemon juice, almond extract, arrowroot, and drained fruit juice; pour over fruit. Mix flour, salt, and baking powder; cut in margarine until mixture is like coarse sugar. Mix egg, nonfat milk, and sweetener; stir into dry ingredients; spoon onto fruit. Bake until browned (25–30 minutes). Serve warm.

MARGARET'S GLAZED BERRY TARTS

Exchanges per serving: 1 filling = ¾ Fruit
                       1 pastry = 1 Starch, 1½ Fat
Calories per serving: filling, 45   Yield: 6 servings
                       pastry, 120

Pastry for 6 medium tarts
1 envelope unflavored
  gelatin
¼ cup cold water
4 cups fresh berries, hulled
  and washed (e.g.,
  strawberries,
  boysenberries)

Nonnutritive sweetener
  equivalent to 1½ cups
  sugar
3 drops food coloring
2 tablespoons lemon juice

Preheat oven to 425°F. Bake tart shells until lightly browned.
Remove from oven; let cool. Soften gelatin in cold water.
Sweeten berries with sweetener and press through strainer until
1½ cups are obtained. Set aside remaining whole berries. Add
coloring and lemon juice; bring to a boil; remove from heat.
Add softened gelatin; stir to dissolve. Chill until mixture begins
to thicken. Arrange remaining whole berries in baked shells.
Cover with gelatin-berry mixture. May be topped with artificial
cream or Low-Calorie Topping Whip (see Index).

YUMMY FRUIT TARTS

Exchanges per serving: 1 filling = ¾ Fat, 1 Fruit,
⅓ Medium-Fat Meat
1 pastry = ⅓ Fat, ¾ Starch
Calories per serving: filling, 105   Yield: 6 tarts
pastry, 76

1 tablespoon arrowroot	1 medium banana, sliced
⅛ teaspoon salt	thin
Nonnutritive sweetener	¼ cup dried coconut,
equivalent to 1 cup sugar	shredded
1 cup fresh orange juice	1 recipe Lorene's Graham
1 cup unsweetened	Cracker Crust (see
pineapple chunks	Index)
2 eggs, beaten	

Combine arrowroot, salt, sweetener, and orange juice. Drain
pineapple, reserving liquid; add sufficient water to make 1 cup.
Combine liquid, arrowroot mixture, and beaten eggs. Cook
over medium heat, stirring constantly, until mixture boils and
thickens; remove from heat. Chill; fold in pineapple chunks,
sliced banana, and coconut. Place in crust; chill until ready
to serve.

CRUMBLY PIECRUST

Exchanges per serving: 1 serving = ⅓ Fat
Calories per serving: 27   Yield: one 9″ crust

3 tablespoons diet	Nonnutritive sweetener
margarine	equivalent to 1
	tablespoon sugar
	¾ cup cornflake crumbs

Preheat oven to 375°F. Mix margarine, sweetener, and crumbs;
press into 9″ pie plate with back of spoon. Press into bottom and
up sides of plate (crust will be fairly thin).

RICH FLAKY CRUST

Exchanges per serving: ⅛ of single piecrust = ¾ Starch, 1½ Fat
Calories per serving: 125 (single crust)   Yield: two 8″ crusts

2 cups flour, sifted   ½ cup oil
1 teaspoon salt   3 tablespoons cold water

Preheat oven to 450°F. Sift flour and salt together; dribble oil on surface; stir with fork until completely mixed. Add cold water to form smooth ball. Divide dough in half. Place half on waxed paper; cover with another piece of waxed paper; roll dough to 12″ circle. Peel off paper; fit into pie plate. For 1-crust pie, flute edges with moistened fork (or finger). Bake until browned (12–15 minutes); cool before filling. For 2-crust pie, place 1 crust (unbaked) into pie plate, put in filling, and top with other crust. Slit upper crust in several places. Bake according to filling instructions. For 2-crust pie, allow 2 Starch and 2 Fat exchanges, and adjust calories to 250 per serving.

PIECRUST

Exchanges per serving: 1 serving = 1 Starch, 1½ Fat
Calories per serving: 120   Yield: one 9″ crust

1⅓ cups flour, sifted   ½ cup diet margarine,
½ teaspoon salt   melted
                               2 tablespoons cold water

Sift flour and salt together; dribble margarine over surface. Stir with fork until completely mixed; add water to margarine-flour mixture; stir to smooth ball. Roll out dough to fit 9″ pie plate. Flute edges with fork. Refrigerate if crust is to be filled prior to baking. If baked unfilled, make several cuts with sharp knife in bottom and sides of crust. Bake at 450°F until golden brown (13–15 minutes).

LORENE'S GRAHAM CRACKER CRUST

Exchanges per serving: 1 serving = ¾ Starch, ⅓ Fat
Calories per serving: 76   Yield: one 9″ crust

1 cup (16) graham crackers, crushed fine	Nonnutritive sweetener equivalent to 2 tablespoons sugar
3 tablespoons diet margarine, melted	

Preheat oven to 350°F. Combine ingredients well; press firmly into a 9″ pie plate. Bake about 10 minutes. Chill before filling.

PASTRY

Exchanges per serving: 1 serving = ¾ Starch, ¾ Fat
Calories per serving: 95   Yield: one 8″ crust

1 cup flour, sifted	5 tablespoons diet margarine
1 teaspoon salt	4 tablespoons water

Preheat oven to 425°F. Combine flour and salt; cut in margarine until consistency of peas. Add water slowly until dough is moistened and holds together. Knead dough lightly, pressing into a ball. Flour pastry board and rolling pin; roll gently, turning often. Roll thin; lay pastry over 8″ pie tin; press down gently, fluting edges. Slit bottom in a few places with sharp knife. Bake until golden brown (about 14–15 minutes). Fill with desired filling. Use extra dough for individual pastries.

CANNING AND FREEZING

CANNING FRUITS

To can fruits, use unsweetened fruit juice or water in place of the usual sugar syrup. Be sure to adhere to processing time and other instructions. When serving, count your fruit exchanges as you would for the commercially prepared sugar-free fruits.

Toss the fruit in lemon juice solution to keep it from darkening. Use sweetener equivalent to 2 to 4 cups of sugar for every 2 to 3 quarts of liquid; if this is not sweet enough (or too sweet), change to suit your taste. The U.S. Department of Agriculture, Washington, DC 20402, has some excellent books on canning that you may wish to send for before trying any recipes.

Use orange or pineapple juice, unsweetened, to obtain an unusual flavor. (These generally settle to the bottom of the jars, so shake well just before serving.) Raspberries and strawberries may be mashed and the juice saved; mixing this juice with water makes an excellent canning liquid.

Apples, grapes, peaches, pears, pineapple, and seedless oranges are fine to mix. A good variation is a half-and-half mixture of peaches and pears. Avoid fruits such as bananas, blueberries, cherries, plums, raspberries, and strawberries in fruit cocktail. (Bananas turn brown and become too soft, while the other fruits "weep" and become too liquid.)

Plums are fine for canning, but be sure you select the proper varieties. Use half water and half plum juice for the canning liquid to help keep the color from being lost.

FREEZING FRUITS WITHOUT SUGAR

Wash and drain thoroughly blackberries, blueberries, cranberries, currants, gooseberries, grapes, pineapple chunks, plums, raspberries, or rhubarb. Leave about ½ inch at top of container when packing. Freeze.

Figs, peaches, and strawberries go into special containers, covered with the ascorbic acid water solution (1 teaspoon crystalline ascorbic acid dissolved in each quart of water). Package, leaving 1 inch at top of quarts and ½ inch for pints. Freeze. Thaw frozen fruits until only a few ice crystals remain and sweeten as desired with nonnutritive sweetener.

VEGETABLES

Nearly any vegetable that can be cooked is recommended for freezing. Order the freezing booklet from the Department of Agriculture, Washington, DC 20402.

CUCUMBER PICKLES

Exchanges per serving: ½ cup = ½ Vegetable
Calories per serving: 13   Yield: 3 pints

6 cucumbers	¼ cup water
¼ cup salt	2 cups white vinegar
Nonnutritive sweetener equivalent to ¾ cup sugar	2 tablespoons pickling spice

Wash and dry cucumbers; cut into strips about 4″ long. Place in large bowl; sprinkle with salt. Let stand overnight. In the morning, rinse and drain well several times. Combine sweetener, water, and vinegar in large pan; bring to boil. Tie pickling spice in cheesecloth bag and add to boiling ingredients. Add cucumbers; reduce heat; simmer about 15 minutes. Place cucumbers in clean hot pint jars. Heat liquid once more to boiling, pour over pickles in jars. Seal immediately.

ANNE'S CHILI SAUCE

Exchanges per serving: 1 tablespoon = 1 free Vegetable
Calories per serving: 6   Yield: 3 quarts

8 cups tomatoes, peeled and chopped
¼ cup red peppers, chopped fine
½ cup green peppers, chopped fine
1½ cups onion, chopped fine
1½ cups celery, chopped fine
Nonnutritive sweetener equivalent to ½ cup sugar
1 tablespoon salt
1½ cups cider vinegar
1 tablespoon Tabasco sauce
1 whole stick cinnamon
1 teaspoon cloves
1½ teaspoons celery seed
1½ teaspoons mustard seed
1 teaspoon Mei Yen seasoning

In a large heavy pan combine first nine ingredients. Combine spices in a cheesecloth bag; add to first mixture. Bring to boil; reduce heat and simmer. Stir occasionally, simmering for about 5–6 hours. Remove bag of spices; pour remainder into clean, hot, pint jars; seal immediately.

JAMS AND JELLIES

JAMS AND JELLIES WITHOUT SUGAR

Cover jars completely with water and bring water to boil. Boil 15 to 20 minutes. Remove jars from water (hold tongs under boiling water 60 to 90 seconds before removing jars so jars do not break); drain jars upside down on aluminum foil until just before using, then turn right side up.

Use your favorite nonnutritive sweetener, being careful to use the proper amount. Stir until it is completely dissolved and mixed. (Do not reboil.)

In top of double boiler, over low heat, melt the paraffin. Pour jams or jellies into jars carefully, and pour on melted paraffin to a thickness of about ¼ inch. Cool. Place in refrigerator. Keep refrigerated, and after first opening, be sure to keep covered with tight lid or aluminum foil molded to top.

APPLE BUTTER JELLY

Exchanges per serving: 1 tablespoon = ¼ Fruit
Calories per serving: 10   Yield: 5¾ cups

8 cups apples, cored, washed, and cut in quarters
2 cups unsweetened apple juice
¼ cup lemon juice
¼ cup cider vinegar
2 teaspoons lemon peel, ground fine
¼ teaspoon nutmeg
1 teaspoon powdered cloves
¼ teaspoon anise seed, ground fine
Nonnutritive sweetener equivalent to ½ cup sugar

Mix all ingredients except sweetener; bring to a boil, stirring constantly; boil a few minutes. Remove from heat, stir in sweetener. Ladle into jelly glasses and seal.

RUTH'S RASPBERRY JAM

Exchanges per serving: 1 tablespoon = Trace Fruit
Calories per serving: 8   Yield: 2 cups

1½ teaspoons unflavored
  gelatin
1½ tablespoons cold water
3 cups fresh raspberries,
  crushed

Nonnutritive sweetener
  equivalent to ⅔ cup
  sugar
¼ teaspoon lemon juice
3 drops red food coloring
  (optional)

Soften gelatin in cold water. Combine berries and sweetener in
saucepan; place on high heat; stir constantly until mixture boils.
Remove from heat; add softened gelatin. Return to heat; cook
for another minute. Remove and blend in lemon juice and food
coloring. Place in pint jar; seal and store in refrigerator.

ANNE'S APPLE JELLY

Exchanges per serving: 1 tablespoon = Trace Fruit
Calories per serving: 10   Yield: 2 cups

2 teaspoons unflavored
  gelatin
2 tablespoons lemon juice
⅛ teaspoon salt
1 teaspoon arrowroot

2 cups apple juice,
  unsweetened
Nonnutritive sweetener
  equivalent to 2 cups
  sugar

Mix gelatin, lemon juice, salt, and arrowroot. Stir in apple juice
and boil, stirring constantly, for two minutes. Remove from
heat; stir in sweetener. Fill jelly jars, seal, and store.

BLUEBERRY JAM

Exchanges per serving: 1 tablespoon = Trace Fruit
Calories per serving: 6   Yield: 2½ cups

2 tablespoons lemon juice	2½ cups frozen
3 tablespoons unflavored	unsweetened blueberries,
gelatin	partially thawed
⅛ teaspoon salt	Nonnutritive sweetener
1½ teaspoons arrowroot	equivalent to 2 cups
	sugar

Mix lemon juice, gelatin, salt, and arrowroot; stir in blueberries.
Boil gently until mixture thickens; stirring constantly (about
3–4 minutes). Stir constantly, boiling at full boil for 2 minutes.
Remove from heat; stir in sweetener. Fill and seal jars.

PHYL'S APPLE JELLY

Exchanges per serving: 1 tablespoon = Trace Fruit
Calories per serving: 10   Yield: 2 cups

4 teaspoons unflavored	Nonnutritive sweetener
gelatin	equivalent to 1 cup sugar
2 cups unsweetened apple	1½ teaspoons lemon juice
juice	3 drops food coloring
	(yellow or green)

Soften gelatin in ½ cup apple juice. Bring the remaining 1½
cups of juice to boil; remove from heat; add softened gelatin.
Stir until gelatin dissolves; add sweetener, lemon juice, and food
coloring. Bring to rolling boil. Place in clean pint jars; seal.
Store in refrigerator.

APPLE-LEMON JELLY

Exchanges per serving: 1 tablespoon = Trace Fruit
Calories per serving: 9   Yield: 2 cups

1 package unflavored gelatin	2 cups apple juice, unsweetened
2 tablespoons lemon juice	Nonnutritive sweetener equivalent to 2 cups sugar
⅛ teaspoon salt	
1 teaspoon arrowroot	

Mix gelatin, lemon juice, salt, and arrowroot; add apple juice and boil, stirring constantly, for two minutes. Remove from heat; add sweetener. Fill prepared jelly jars; seal.

STRAWBERRY JELLY

Exchanges per serving: 1 tablespoon = Trace Fruit
Calories per serving: 5   Yield: 5½ cups

2 envelopes unflavored gelatin	4 cups strawberries, hulled, washed, and strained
½ cup lemon juice	Nonnutritive sweetener equivalent to 4 cups sugar
Dash of salt	
1 tablespoon arrowroot	

Mix gelatin, lemon juice, salt, and arrowroot; add strawberries. Boil, stirring constantly, about 3 minutes. Remove from heat; stir in sweetener. Fill and seal jars.

PINEAPPLE-APRICOT JAM

Exchanges per serving: 1 tablespoon = ¼ Fruit
Calories per serving: 15   Yield: 5 cups

2 cups dried apricots	2 tablespoons lemon juice
2 cups water	Dash of salt
4 cups unsweetened pineapple tidbits	Nonnutritive sweetener equivalent to 1 cup sugar

Boil apricots in water until tender (about 25 minutes). Drain pineapple tidbits and cut each one in half. Puree apricots and water with lemon juice and salt. Return to saucepan; stir in pineapple. Boil a few minutes, stirring now and then. Remove from heat; add sweetener. Fill jelly jars; seal.

CONSERVE

Exchanges per serving: 1 tablespoon = ⅙ Fat, ¼ Fruit
Calories per serving: 22   Yield: 2 cups

1 cup dried apricots	2 tablespoons lemon juice
2 cups water	Nonnutritive sweetener
2¼ cups unsweetened	equivalent to 1 cup sugar
pineapple tidbits	½ cup nuts, finely chopped
⅛ teaspoon salt	

Boil apricots in water until tender; puree. Drain pineapple tidbits; cut each piece into smaller pieces. Put apricot puree in saucepan; add pineapple, salt, and lemon juice. Boil slowly, stirring constantly, about 5 minutes. Remove from heat; stir in sweetener and nuts. Fill jars; seal.

JOAN'S CHUTNEY

Exchanges per serving: ¼ cup = 1 Fruit
Calories per serving: 45   Yield: 1½ pints

¾ cup white raisins
¼ cup bell peppers, chopped fine
1 cup white vinegar
4 pears, cored, pared, and chopped

Nonnutritive sweetener equivalent to 2 cups sugar
½ teaspoon ginger
¼ teaspoon allspice
¼ teaspoon cloves
¼ teaspoon salt

Combine all ingredients in large pan; bring to boil. Reduce heat to medium; cook until pears are tender and mixture is slightly thick (about an hour). Spoon into 3 clear ½-pint jars and seal immediately.

CONVERTING THESE RECIPES FOR MICROWAVE OVENS

When you've found a recipe in our book you would like to use, try to find a similar one in your microwave recipe book. The amounts of ingredients in these recipes should match the ingredients in the microwave recipe. Make sure the dish is recommended for microwave cooking and is similar in size, shape, and cooking temperature.

Compare the corresponding cooking method and be sure you follow all directions carefully—including directions for covering the dish or not and whether waxed paper or plastic wrap is to be used in any covering.

Refer to general information on food categories for each ingredient in your microwave cookbook. Also check the charts for meats and vegetables, suggested cooking times, and weights.

Certain types of food vary in cooking times: bread has very little moisture content, while vegetables have more moisture content and require longer times; potatoes and eggs whites, which have little sugar or fat, take longer to cook than such foods as egg yolks and certain fruits, because the latter contain a greater amount of fat or sugar.

Be sure foods cooked in the microwave oven are not overcooked. Check them frequently. When you first try converting recipes, you will have to experiment. Allow for extra time to prepare these recipes.

Remember that the foods continue to cook once they are removed from the microwave oven, so remove them at the correct time. This is usually 10 to 20 minutes for meat and 5 to 10 minutes for vegetables.

It may be necessary to decrease the amount of liquid or increase the thickening agent in the diabetic recipes, as liquids evaporate more slowly in a microwave oven. You may also need to adjust the liquid if the recipe calls for short cooking time.

Lack of evaporation intensifies flavors, so it is generally best to add herbs, seasonings, and spices by taste after cooking, or else reduce amounts you'd usually use. Salt, in particular, should be added *last*, as it draws out moisture in the foods when microwaved. (Meat and vegetables should *not* be salted until cooking is finished.) Cloves, garlic, garlic powder, onion, and other seasoning blends may be used in lieu of salt and will not have the drying effect of salt.

Because there is a lack of dry heat source, breads (quick and yeast), cakes, and cookies develop in a unique way—they are fluffier since they are not restricted by a crust. As steam rises to the surface after cooking, the tops of cakes will be moist and wet-looking. They will toughen if you overcook, as this removes the moist appearance from these baked goods. With the exception of chocolate, baked products will be pale and not crusty. We suggest using about ½ the amount of baking powder and soda when you are adapting one of our recipes for microwaving. To help prevent an irregular-shaped top, a lower power setting is preferable. It's best to use recipes for cookies that do not need browning and are soft, such as bars, etc. We do not suggest baking angel food and chiffon cakes in the microwave.

Following are some microwave conversion examples.

MEATLOAF

Regular recipe:

1 egg

2 cups ground beef (lean)

3 slices bread, cubed fine

¼ cup catsup (see Index)

⅓ cup onion, chopped fine

Conversion:

1 pound lean ground beef

2 slices white bread (day old) cubed

3 tablespoons milk

2 tablespoons finely chopped onion

1 egg

2 teaspoons Worcestershire sauce

½ teaspoon salt

Dash of pepper

Preheat oven to 400°F. Mix all ingredients well. Form into loaf. Place in 9″ × 5″ pan; bake until done (15–20 minutes).

Combine all ingredients. Spread in 9″ × 5″ ungreased glass or ceramic loaf dish. Microwave at High 17–21 minutes, or until center is firm and meat has lost its pink color (internal temperature 145–150°F). Rotate dish after half the cooking time. Let stand 5–10 minutes.

CRUMB CRUST

1 cup (16) graham
   crackers, crushed fine
3 tablespoons diet
   margarine, melted
Nonnutritive sweetener
   equivalent to 2
   tablespoons sugar

Preheat oven to 350°F. Combine ingredients well; press firmly into a 9″ pie plate. Bake about 10 minutes. Chill before filling.

To adapt to microwaving without changing ingredients: Use graham crackers, chocolate or vanilla wafers, or ginger snaps. Melt margarine in 9″ glass or ceramic pie plate. Stir in crumbs and sweetener, if used. Press firmly against bottom and sides of plate using another pie plate or a ramekin to press evenly in pie plate. Microwave 1½ minutes, turning after 1 minute. Let cool before filling.

HINTS AND TIPS FOR MICROWAVING

Selecting Recipes for Conversion

It's best to start with a familiar recipe while you're learning conversion techniques. It helps to adapt it for microwaving when you know how the food is supposed to look and taste. Make sure the flavors and the proportions seem pleasing if you have not yet tried our recipe.

Then check the list of foods that won't work! (See your own microwave oven cookbook.) Can you achieve the cooking technique by microwaving?

Microwaving is a natural for moist cooking—check for recipes that call for covering, liquid, or steaming as this shows the food needs moisture and should do well in the microwave. It is much more satisfactory to use a conventional oven if a crust or dry surface is essential to the recipe.

Some foods may be slightly different when microwaved even though they can be adapted. Cakes will be more tender, omelets won't brown or have a crust—but you may even prefer the microwave version.

To help foods microwave evenly, stir or turn foods over. Recipes should adapt easily if our recipe allows for stirring or turning. Can you include stirring in a microwave recipe if ours does not call for stirring? Yes, rotate the dish and reduce the power setting if the recipe would be changed by too much stirring.

Select a recipe in your microwave cookbook with the same quality and quantity of main bulky ingredients, and a similar amount and type of liquid. (Liquid may be either like chicken broth, which you can microwave at "high," or delicate, like cream, which may take a lower power setting.)

Cubed sirloin is a higher quality meat that is microwaved in a different way than cubed chuck, as chuck is a less tender cut.

More food takes more time, so quantity is important. Follow the conversion guidelines; but if our recipe calls for a different amount of food, you will need to adjust the cooking time.

Substituting Ingredients

You can generally make the same substitutions you ordinarily use for any of our recipes. For instance, if you prefer to use dried onions rather than fresh, follow directions on the package and use them in microwaving. Most seasonings are interchangeable—you can substitute any herb you like, in any recipe, for one you may not care for. Some substitutions—such as using processed cheeses, which melt more smoothly, instead of dry or hard natural cheeses—are recommended for microwaving. "Quick-cooking" rice can be substituted for raw or converted rice; in the short time it takes to microwave the other ingredients in your casserole, the rice will be tender.

But you should be more careful with those substitutions that affect the microwaving times, method, or power setting.

You may need medium or a lower power, and double the time, if you substitute cream for milk. If using converted rice rather than quick-cooking rice, be sure to microwave the rice until partially tender before adding other ingredients. If flour is used in lieu of cornstarch in a sauce, increase amount as you would normally do and stir the sauce more frequently.

The consistency of a dish may be affected by some substitutions. If you are using yogurt rather than sour cream, reduce the amount because yogurt is more liquid.

Selecting the Microwave Method for One of Our Recipes

You can achieve most of the cooking methods called for in these recipes by microwaving.

Don't try deep-frying! This and boiling are the two conventional cooking methods that cannot be achieved with microwaving.

1. **TO OVEN BAKE:** Preheat oven and cook foods, covered or uncovered, at recommended temperature. If steam is desired, place a pan of water in oven.

   TO MICROWAVE BAKE: Using recommended power setting, microwave food, covered or uncovered. (Never preheat oven.)

2. **TO BRAISE, CASSEROLE, ROAST, STEW:** Sometimes fruit, meat, and vegetables are browned first, then simmered in liquid in a covered pan, generally on top of range or in oven. Stew takes more liquid than braising. Casseroles and roasted meats don't need additional liquid as they are cooked on a bed of moist vegetables.

   TO MICROWAVE BRAISE, CASSEROLE, ROAST, STEW: Do not brown; reduce amount of liquid. Use a cooking bag or cover tightly and microwave at "medium" or "medium low."

3. **TO PAN-BROIL OR PAN-FRY:** Cook food uncovered to keep crisp and dry. For pan-broiling, do not use fat; use a small amount of fat for pan-frying.

TO MICROWAVE PAN-BROIL OR PAN-FRY: Follow directions for preheating browning utensil. If broiling, add no fat; if pan-frying add fat. Microwave food, uncovered, on both sides.

4. **TO POACH:** Chicken, eggs, fish, and fruit are gently simmered in liquid to cover.

TO MICROWAVE POACH: To produce steam, reduce liquid to 1 cup or less. Using plastic wrap, tightly cover dish. The type of food will determine power setting.

5. **TO ROAST:** Elevate meat on a rack placed in a shallow pan. Cook uncovered to desired internal temperature, basting occasionally to keep surface moist.

TO MICROWAVE ROAST: Meat should be placed on a rack in uncovered baking dish. Turn meat over after half the cooking time, but it is not necessary to baste. Microwave at "medium" or "medium-low," using probe or microwave thermometer.

6. **TO SAUTÉ:** Brown or sear food in butter or oil. Cover and simmer over low heat. Add small amount of liquid or moist vegetables to chicken or meat.

TO MICROWAVE SAUTÉ: Unless desired for flavoring, omit fat and browning. Find the proper power setting suitable for the food and microwave, covered.

7. **TO STEAM:** Set a rack over boiling water and place food on it, or surround container of food with simmering water, in covered pot. Do not allow water to touch food in either case.

TO MICROWAVE STEAM: Microwave moist foods in a tightly covered dish. Do not use water. If cooking delicate foods, such as mousse, place the mold in a dish of hot water and microwave uncovered.

8. **TO STIR-FRY:** Using a small amount of oil, fry small pieces of food quickly. Stir constantly to prevent sticking. Add quick-cooking foods last; if desired, add sauce.

   TO MICROWAVE STIR-FRY: Follow directions for preheating browning dish. Add oil and long-cooking foods. Stir every 2 minutes. Add quick-cooking foods last. If desired, add sauce.

Testing and Timing Microwave Recipes for Doneness

Cooking time is the major difference between these recipes and the microwave adaptation. Check your microwave oven for wattage. If yours has a very high wattage, check to see if your food is done *before* the minimum time. Varying speed and evenness of cooking are found in different microwave ovens. Some may be slower with heavy or light loads, and some operate more efficiently with a medium food load. The cookbook you received with your own microwave oven will help you in estimating minimum and/or maximum times. It is possible your book may recommend stirring or turning more frequently—good results may depend on the extra attention suggested.

Unless the food is one that needs more time to rehydrate or tenderize, generally the microwaving time will be approximately a fourth to a half of the conventional time. Don't believe that in microwaving a few seconds' difference can ruin the food. Cooking times help you *estimate* how long the food may take in both conventional and microwaving ovens, but *you* are the final judge of when it is done.

1. **ADD:** If you see it is needed to match consistency of our recipe, add a little more liquid.

2. **DON'T ADD:** Be sure you reduce salt and DO NOT add until recipe is done.

3. **SCALE:** To help estimate cooking time according to weight of food and power setting, a microwave scale is a very useful tool.

4. **STIR:** If food seems to be cooking unevenly, rotate the dish or turn the food.

5. **TASTE:** When cooking is completed, especially the first time you convert a recipe, taste! (This is also a big help in judging consistency, tenderness, and texture.)

6. **TEST:** Doneness tests are, for most recipes, the same for conventional ovens as for microwave ovens. Check for doneness at the minimum time; overcooking is a real problem, and you can always cook longer! Don't forget to allow for standing time when required.

7. **WATCH:** Frequently check the progress of cooking. It does not harm the food to interrupt the cooking.

CONVECTION OVENS

Makers say that cooking in shorter periods and at lower temperatures are the advantages to the convection ovens. The fan blows hot air around foods and the air circulation cooks on all exposed sides. These are not as good as regular ovens in every category of food, for quality, in our opinion, but you can use any recipe in our book in one of the convection ovens. Be sure you watch the food so it is not cooked too rapidly. You must experiment with any new oven and this is no exception!

HOW TO USE NUTRITION LABELING TO WORK OUT FOOD EXCHANGES

Most foods are now labeled with carbohydrate, fat, and protein information. We felt the following material would be most helpful.

This method was developed by the Diabetes Education Center, Minneapolis, MN, and is made available through the cooperation and courtesy of The Pillsbury Company and in particular Ms. Suzanne J. Carlson, Pillsbury Department of Nutrition.

FOOD EXCHANGES USING NUTRITION LABELING

This method uses the Exchange List for Meal Planning developed by the American Diabetes Association, Inc., and The American Dietetic Association, and is offered here through the courtesy of The Pillsbury Company. Should you have questions about using the following Exchange List, consult your dietition or physician.

Food products now carry nutrition labeling on the package. This nutrition information makes it possible for diabetics to include many more foods in their diets, using the method that is described here.

Any company that uses nutrition labeling must follow the format set out by the FDA. This is the part of the information you need to work out the exchanges.

One 10″ Cheese Pizza Nutrition Information per Serving	
Serving size	½ pizza
Servings per container	2
Calories per serving	438
Protein	22 grams
Carbohydrates	52 grams
Fat	16 grams

How to Work Out Food Exchanges

You need this exchange list for reference:

Exchange	Calories*	Carbo-hydrate	Protein	Fat
1 Milk (Skim) Exchange	90	12 grams	8 grams	trace
1 Vegetable Exchange	25	5 grams	2 grams	—
1 Fruit Exchange	60	15 grams	—	—
1 Starch Exchange	80	15 grams	3 grams	0–1 gram
1 Meat Exchange, Very Lean Meat	35	—	7 grams	0-1 gram
Lean	55	—	7 grams	3 grams
Medium-Fat	75	—	7 grams	5 grams
High-Fat	100	—	7 grams	8 grams
1 Fat Exchange	45	—	—	5 grams

We will use the pizza label shown before as an example. With practice, this method can be used for other food products with nutrition labeling and used for various serving sizes of a product. You need this information from the nutrition label:

Serving size	½ pizza
Servings per container	2
Calories per serving	438
Protein	22 grams
Carbohydrates	52 grams
Fat	16 grams

* Carbohydrate and protein provide 4 calories/gm; fat provides 9 calories/gm.

	Exchanges	Carbo-hydrate	Protein	Fat
1. List the grams of carbohydrate, protein, and fat from pizza label.		52	22	16
2. Divide the carbohydrate (52 gm) by 15 gm to get the number of Starch Exchanges (52 ÷ 15 = 37/15, which is rounded to 3 Starch Exchanges*) List the carbohydrate, protein, and fat in the 3 Starch Exchanges.	Starch—3	−45	−9	0
		7	13	16
Subtract from label values.				
3. Divide the remaining carbohydrate (7) by 5 gm to get the number of Vegetable Exchanges.** List the carbohydrate, protein, and fat values for the Vegetable Exchange.	Veg.—1	−5	−2	0
		2	11	16
Subtract from label values.				
4. Divide the remaining protein (11) by 7 gm to get the number of Meat Exchanges.	Medium-Fat Meat 1½			

* Carbohydrate and protein provide 4 calories/gm; fat provides 9 calories/gm.
** Count whole and nearest ½ exchanges; disregard less.

List the carbohydrate,
protein, and fat values
for Meat Exchanges.

$$\frac{0}{2} \quad \frac{-11}{0} \frac{-7.5}{8.5}$$

Subtract from label values.

5. Divide the remaining
   fat (8.5) by 5 gm to
   get the Fat Exchange.   Fat—1½

$$\frac{0}{2} \quad \frac{0}{0} \frac{-8.5}{0}$$

List and subtract.

	Carbo-hydrate	Protein	Fat	Calories
6. Therefore, one serving of pizza is equivalent to 3 Starch, 1 Vegetable, 1½ Medium-Fat Meat and 1½ Fat Exchanges.				
7. As a final check, ½ pizza Exchanges (3 Starch, 1 Vegetable, 1½ Meat, and 1½ Fat).	52 gm	22 gm	16 gm	428
	50 gm	22 gm	16 gm	445

FOOD BUYING GUIDE FOR FRUITS AND VEGETABLES

The following chart is from the August 1979 "National Consumer Buying Alert," a publication of The White House, Office of Special Assistant for Consumer Affairs.

Storage and cooking properly can maximize your nutrient intake from both fruit and vegetables. The chart lists nutrients contained in common fruit and vegetables and gives tips for storing, including the lapse of time before eating quality is affected. Serving yield per pound or piece(s) is also provided. As you will note in our Fruit and Vegetable Exchange Lists, one serving usually equals approximately ½ cup, 1 medium, or 2 small fruits.

Use as little water or liquid as possible to better preserve the nutrients in cooking. (Steaming vegetables on a rack with water under the rack is a fine way to retain food values.) Another nutrient-preserving way to cook potatoes and other root vegetables that are high in water content is in a microwave oven without water.

Product	Nutrients*	Storage Tips	For Best Eating Quality Use Within**	Servings per Unit***
Fresh Vegetables				
Asparagus	Vitamins C and A, iron	Refrigerate in crisper or in plastic bags.	2 or 3 days	2 or 3 per pound
Beans, lima	Iron, B vitamins, fiber	Store uncovered in pods in refrigerator.	3 to 5 days	2 or 3 per pound

Product	Nutrients*	Storage Tips	For Best Eating Quality Use Within**	Servings per Unit***
Beans, snap	Iron, fiber	Refrigerate in crisper or in plastic bags.	1 week	5 or 6 per pound
Beets	Fiber	Refrigerate in crisper or in plastic bags; remove tops before storing.	2 weeks	3 or 4 per pound
Broccoli	Vitamin A, B vitamins, vitamin C, iron, magnesium, fiber	Refrigerate in crisper or in plastic bags.	3 to 5 days	5 or 6 per pound
Brussels sprouts	Vitamin C, B vitamins, iron, magnesium, fiber	Refrigerate in crisper or in plastic bags.	3 to 5 days	5 or 6 per pound
Cabbage	Vitamin C, fiber	Refrigerate in crisper or in plastic bags.	1 or 2 weeks	11 or 12 per pound (shredded) 4 to 5 per pound (cooked)

Product	Nutrients*	Storage Tips	For Best Eating Quality Use Within**	Servings per Unit***
Carrots	Vitamin A, fiber	Refrigerate in crisper or in plastic bags; remove tops before storing.	2 weeks	5 or 6 per pound
Cauliflower	Vitamin C, fiber	Refrigerate in crisper or in plastic bags.	1 week	6 (raw) 5 (cooked)
Celery	Fiber	Refrigerate in crisper or in plastic bags; dry thoroughly if washed before storing.	1 week	3 (raw) 6 to 7 (cooked)
Corn	Fiber	Store unhusked and uncovered in refrigerator.	1 or 2 days	1 per ear
Cucumbers	—	Refrigerate in crisper or in plastic bags.	1 week	5

Product	Nutrients*	Storage Tips	For Best Eating Quality Use Within**	Servings per Unit***
Greens (kale, collards, etc.)	Vitamin A, B vitamins, vitamin C, calcium, iron, magnesium, fiber	Refrigerate in crisper or in plastic bags; dry thoroughly if washed before storing.	3 to 5 days	6
Lettuce	—	Refrigerate in crisper or in plastic bags; dry thoroughly if washed before storing.	1 week	6 to 8 cups shredded per pound
Mushrooms	Fiber	Refrigerate in crisper or in plastic bags.	1 or 2 days	9 (raw) 4 (cooked)
Okra	Vitamin C, fiber	Refrigerate in crisper or in plastic bags.	3 to 5 days	5
Onions, green	—	Refrigerate in crisper or in plastic bags.	3 to 5 days	4 to 6 per bunch
Onions	—	Store in cool (60°F), dry place.	Several months	3 to 4—cooked

Product	Nutrients*	Storage Tips	For Best Eating Quality Use Within**	Servings per Unit***
Peas, green (in pods)	B vitamins, iron, fiber	Store uncovered in pods in refrigerator.	3 to 5 days	2
Potatoes	Vitamin C, B vitamins, fiber	Store in dry dark place (45°–50°F). Note that potatoes will lose vitamin C gradually over a period of several months.	Several months	3 or 4 per pound
Radishes	—	Refrigerate in crisper or in plastic bags; remove tops before storing.	2 weeks	6
Spinach	Vitamin A, B vitamins, vitamin C, calcium, iron, magnesium, fiber	Refrigerate in crisper or in plastic bags; dry thoroughly if washed before storing.	3 to 5 days	6

Product	Nutrients*	Storage Tips	For Best Eating Quality Use Within**	Servings per Unit***
Squash, summer	Fiber, vitamin A	Refrigerate in crisper or in plastic bags.	3 to 5 days	4
Fresh Fruits				
Apples	Fiber	Wash and dry, then refrigerate.	Few weeks	3 or 4 per pound
Apricots	Vitamin A, fiber	Wash and dry, then refrigerate.	3 to 5 days	5 or 6 per pound
Bananas	B vitamins, magnesium, fiber	Ripen at room temperature. Store in refrigerator. Skin will darken, but flesh will remain flavorful and firm.	3 to 5 days	3 or 4 per pound

Product	Nutrients*	Storage Tips	For Best Eating Quality Use Within**	Servings per Unit***
Blueberries	Iron, fiber	Do not wash before storing. Refrigerate—leave on stems and store loosely in shallow container so air can circulate and bottom fruits are not crushed.	3 to 5 days	3 or 4 per pint
Cherries	Vitamin C	Do not wash before storing. Refrigerate—leave on stems and store loosely in shallow container so air can circulate and bottom fruits are not crushed.	1 or 2 days	5 or 6 per pound
Grapefruit	Vitamin C	Store at cool room temperature.	2 weeks	2 per fruit

Product	Nutrients*	Storage Tips	For Best Eating Quality Use Within**	Servings per Unit***
Grapes	Vitamin C	Refrigerate—will not ripen further after picking, so choose ripe fruit.	3 to 5 days	5 or 6 per pound
Nectarines	Vitamin A, fiber	Wash and dry, then refrigerate.	3 to 5 days	3 or 4 per pound
Oranges	Vitamin C, fiber	Store at cool room temperature.	2 weeks	3 to 4 per pound
Peaches	Vitamin A, fiber	Wash and dry, then refrigerate.	3 to 5 days	3 or 4 per pound
Pears	Fiber	Wash and dry, then refrigerate.	3 to 5 days	3 or 4 per pound
Pineapple	—	Wash and dry, then refrigerate. Will not ripen further after picking, so select ripe fruit.	1 or 2 days	6 to 8 per fruit

Product	Nutrients*	Storage Tips	For Best Eating Quality Use Within**	Servings per Unit***
Plums	Vitamin C, fiber	Wash and dry, then refrigerate.	3 to 5 days	3 to 4 per pound
Raspberries	Vitamin C, iron, fiber	Do not wash before storing. Refrigerate—leave on stems and store loosely in shallow container so air can circulate and bottom fruits are not crushed	1 or 2 days	4 to 5 per pint
Strawberries	Vitamin C, iron, fiber	Do not wash before storing. Refrigerate—leave on stems and store loosely in shallow container so air can circulate and bottom fruits are not crushed.	1 or 2 days	3 to 4 per pint

Product	Nutrients*	Storage Tips	For Best Eating Quality Use Within**	Servings per Unit***
Watermelon	Vitamin C	Wash and dry, then refrigerate. Will not ripen further after picking, so shop for ripe fruit.	3 to 5 days	10 or more depending on size

* Most fruits and vegetables contain no cholesterol and little or no fat. Most vegetables provide less than 50 Calories per serving. Starchy vegetables—corn, lima beans, peas, and potatoes—provide less than 100 calories per serving. (See Fruits and Vegetables Lists for accurate amounts.)

** Storage time is longer for unripened fruits and vegetables, but once ripe, these numbers apply.

*** One serving equals approximately ½ cup, 1 medium-size fruit, 2 small fruits, or ½ banana.

RECOMMENDED DIETARY ALLOWANCES, REVISED 1995

Designed for the maintenance of good nutrition of practically all healthy people in the United States of America. Food and Nutrition Board, National Academy of Sciences–National Research Council.

Age (YR)	Weight (kg)	Weight (lb)	Height (cm)	Height (inches)	ENERGY (kcal)	PROTEIN (g)	VITAMIN A (µg RE)	VITAMIN D (µg)	VITAMIN E (mg or TE)	VITAMIN K (µg)	VITAMIN C (mg)	THIAMIN (mg)	RIBOFLAVIN (mg)	NIACIN (mg NE)	VITAMIN B₆ (mg)	FOLATE (µg)	VITAMIN B₁₂ (µg)	CALCIUM (mg)	PHOSPHORUS (mg)	MAGNESIUM (mg)	IRON (mg)	ZINC (mg)	IODINE (µg)	SELENIUM (µg)
Infants																								
0.0–0.5	6	13	60	24	650	13	375	7.5	3	5	30	0.3	0.4	5	0.3	25	0.3	400	300	40	6	5	40	10
0.5–1.0	9	20	71	28	850	14	375	10	4	10	35	0.4	0.3	6	0.6	35	0.5	600	500	60	10	5	50	15
Children																								
1–3	13	29	90	35	1300	16	400	10	6	15	40	0.7	0.8	9	1.0	50	0.7	800	800	80	10	10	70	20
4–6	20	44	112	44	1800	24	500	10	7	20	45	0.9	1.1	12	1.1	75	1.0	800	800	120	10	10	90	20
7–10	28	62	132	57	2000	28	700	10	7	30	45	1.0	1.2	13	1.4	100	1.4	800	800	170	10	10	120	30
Males																								
11–14	45	99	157	62	2500	45	1000	10	10	45	50	1.3	1.5	17	1.7	150	2.0	1200	1200	270	12	15	150	40
15–18	66	145	176	69	3000	59	1000	10	10	65	60	1.5	1.8	20	2.0	200	2.0	1200	1200	400	12	15	150	50

Age (YR)	Weight (kg)	Weight (lb)	Height (cm)	Height (inches)	ENERGY (kcal)	PROTEIN (g)	VITAMIN A (µg RE)	VITAMIN D (µg)	VITAMIN E (mg or TE)	VITAMIN K (µg)	VITAMIN C (mg)	THIAMIN (mg)	RIBOFLAVIN (mg)	NIACIN (mg NE)	VITAMIN B6 (mg)	FOLATE (µg)	VITAMIN B12 (µg)	CALCIUM (mg)	PHOSPHORUS (mg)	MAGNESIUM (mg)	IRON (mg)	ZINC (mg)	IODINE (µg)	SELENIUM (µg)
19–24	72	160	177	70	2900	58	1000	10	10	70	60	1.5	1.7	19	2.0	200	2.0	1200	1200	350	10	15	150	70
25–50	79	174	176	70	2900	63	1000	5	10	80	60	1.5	1.7	19	2.0	200	2.0	800	800	350	10	15	150	70
51+	77	170	173	68	2300	63	1000	5	10	80	60	1.2	1.4	15	2.0	200	2.0	800	800	350	10	15	150	70
Females																								
11–14	46	101	157	62	2200	46	800	10	8	45	50	1.1	1.3	15	1.4	150	2.0	1200	1200	280	15	12	150	45
15–18	55	120	163	64	2200	44	800	10	8	55	60	1.1	1.3	15	1.5	180	2.0	1200	1200	300	15	12	150	50
19–24	58	128	164	65	2200	46	800	10	8	60	60	1.1	1.3	15	1.6	180	2.0	1200	1200	280	15	12	150	55
25–50	63	138	163	64	2200	50	800	5	8	65	60	1.1	1.3	15	1.6	180	2.0	800	800	280	15	12	150	55
51+	65	143	160	63	1900	50	800	5	8	65	60	1.0	1.2	13	1.6	180	2.0	800	800	280	10	12	150	55
Pregnant					+300	60	800	10	10	65	70	1.5	1.6	17	2.2	400	2.2	1200	1200	320	30	15	175	65
Lactating																								
1st 6 mo.					+500	65	1300	10	12	65	95	1.6	1.8	20	2.1	280	2.6	1200	1200	355	15	19	200	75
2nd. 6 mo.					+500	62	1200	10	11	65	90	1.6	1.7	20	2.1	260	2.6	1200	1200	340	15	16	200	75

Estimated safe and adequate daily dietary intakes of additional selected vitamins and minerals.*

age group	vitamins			trace elements**		
	vitamin K	biotin	pantothenic acid	copper	manganese	fluoride
	← µg →		← mg →			
infants						
0.0–0.5 yr.	12	35	2	0.5–0.7	0.5–0.7	0.1–0.5
0.5–1.0 yr.	10–20	50	3	0.7–1.0	0.7–1.0	0.2–1.0
children and adolescents						
1–3 yr.	15–30	65	3	1.0–1.5	1.0–1.5	0.5–1.5
4–6 yr.	20–40	85	3–4	1.5–2.0	1.5–2.0	1.0–2.5
7–10 yr.	30–60	120	4–5	2.0–2.5	2.0–3.0	1.5–2.5
11+ yr.	50–100	100–200	4–7	2.0–3.0	2.5–5.0	1.5–2.5
adults	70–140	100–200	4–7	2.0–3.0	2.5–5.0	1.5–4.0

trace elements**			electrolytes		
chromium	selenium	molybdenum	sodium	potassium	chloride
←			_mg_		→
0.01–0.04	0.01–0.04	0.03–0.06	115–350	350–925	275–700
0.02–0.06	0.02–0.06	0.04–0.08	250–750	425–1,275	400–1,200
0.02–0.08	0.02–0.08	0.05–0.1	325–975	550–1,650	500–1,500
0.03–0.12	0.03–0.12	0.06–0.15	450–1,350	775–2,325	700–2,100
0.05–0.2	0.05–0.2	0.1–0.3	600–1,800	1,000–3,000	925–2,775
0.05–0.2	0.05–0.2	0.15–0.5	900–2,700	1,525–4,575	1,400–4,200
0.05–0.2	0.05–0.2	0.15–0.5	1,100–3,300	1,875–5,625	1,700–5,100

* From Recommended Dietary Allowances. Revised 1980. Food and Nutrition Board, National Academy of Sciences–National Research Council. Because there is less information on which to base allowances, these figures are not given in the main table of the RDAs and are provided here in the form of ranges of recommended intakes.

** Since the toxic levels for many trace elements may be only several times usual intakes, the upper levels for the trace elements given in this table should not be habitually exceeded.

PRINTED MATERIAL AVAILABLE

For information, we suggest that you write to the following:

American Diabetes Association
1660 Duke Street
Alexandria, VA 22314

Juvenile Diabetes Foundation
23 East 26th Street
New York, NY 10010

The American Dietetic
  Association
216 W. Jackson Blvd., Suite 700
Chicago, IL 60606-6995

Recommended by the U.S. Department of Health and Human Services, Public Health Service, and the National Institute of Health is a booklet called "How to Cope with Diabetes," prepared by the National Institute of Arthritis, Metabolism, and Digestive Diseases, Bethesda, MD 20014.

"Family Cookbooks, Vols. I, II, and III" are available for $16.95 plus S/H. For information on how to order, contact either:

American Diabetes Assoc.
Order Dept.
1660 Duke Street
Alexandria, VA 22314

or:

The American Dietetic Assoc.
216 W. Jackson Blvd.
Suite 700
Chicago, IL 60606-6995

Many drug companies that sell products intended for diabetes offer excellent publications on diabetes free of charge. They will gladly forward information upon request. Among these are:

Ames Company
Division of Miles
  Laboratories, Inc.
Elkhart, IN 46514

Guidebook for the Diabetic Patient,
  Mr. Hypo is My Friend (a cartoon book for the education of preschool diabetics), and a diabetes identification key chain.

DIABETES RESEARCH AND TRAINING CENTERS

Dr. Norman S. Fleischer
Albert Einstein College of
  Medicine
1300 Morris Park Avenue
Bronx, NY 10461
(212) 430-2908

Dr. Stefan Fajans
Endocrinology & Metabolism
  Division
University of Michigan
School of Medicine
Ann Arbor, MI 58104
(734) 764-4165, or 647-5888
  (admin.)

Dr. Arthur H. Rubenstein
Diabetes Research & Training
  Center
University of Chicago
950 East 59th Street
Chicago, IL 60637
(773) 947-5536

Dr. Steve Davis
Diabetes Research & Training
  Center
Vanderbilt University
School of Medicine
Nashville, TN 37232
(615) 322-2197

Dr. Charles M. Clark, Jr.
Department of Medicine
Indiana University Medical
  Center
1100 West Michigan Street
Indianapolis, IN 46202
(317) 554-0000 (x2266 or 2267)

Dr. William H. Daughaday
Washington University Diabetes
  Research & Training Center
660 South Euclid
St. Louis, MO 63110
(314) 935-5000

Dr. George Cahill
Joslin Diabetes Foundation, Inc.
1 Joslin Place
Boston, MA 02215
(617) 732-2541, or 732-2565
  (admin.)

Dr. Joseph Larner
Diabetes Research & Training
  Center
University of Virginia
Charlottesville, VA 22903
(804) 924-2321, or 924-5860
  (admin.)

DIABETES-ENDOCRINOLOGY
RESEARCH CENTERS

Dr. Franz Matschinsky
Diabetes-Endocrinology Center
University of Pennsylvania
School of Medicine
Philadelphia, PA 19104
(215) 622-3165

Dr. Daryl K. Granner
Professor of Medicine and
  Biochemistry
Department of Internal
  Medicine
College of Medicine
University of Iowa
Iowa City, IA 52242

Dr. Daniel Ports, Jr.
Diabetes-Endocrinology
  Center
University of Washington
1131 Fourteenth Avenue South,
  at R8
Seattle, WA 98195
(206) 762-1010 (x493)

Index

Page numbers in bold indicate tables.

Author's Note

I have written this book because many diabetics have expressed their desire for a cookbook with recipes and helpful suggestions specifically related to their dietary needs.

This collection offers a large variety of unusual and basic recipes that have been kitchen tested and used for hospital patients on diabetic diets. Any of these recipes may be adapted for general use by substituting the equivalent amount of regular sugar for the artificial noncaloric sugar substitutes. Where ingredients you are unable to tolerate are called for, you can usually omit them; the finished product may perhaps be a bit less tasty, but it can probably be eaten with enjoyment just the same.

The caloric content and the exchange-group breakdown for each measured individual serving have been carefully calculated. There are helpful hints for using diet ingredients, for restaurant dining, and for preparation of box lunches. We have also included reference materials—tables of weights and measures (including metric tables), weight tables, diabetic exchange lists (with a special table of packaged foods), tables of nutrient values of foods, aids to varying meals, and daily menu guides.

Cookbooks have been published to assist diabetics, but to my knowledge, the subject has not been approached elsewhere from so comprehensive a point of view.

I had you all in mind while writing this, and I hope it will become the most useful book on your cookbook shelf.

Billie Little
(with appreciation to
Sally Murphy)